Turn these pages at your own risk.
Chew each paragraph at least fifty times.
Relax and enjoy.

—William Dufty

# MICHIO KUSHI
# ON THE GREATER VIEW

**Collected Thoughts and Ideas on Macrobiotics and Humanity**

# MICHIO KUSHI ON

## Collected Thoughts and Ideas

# THE GREATER VIEW

## on Macrobiotics and Humanity

Compiled by the Editors of
## the East West Journal

AVERY PUBLISHING GROUP INC.
Wayne, New Jersey

The therapeutic procedures in this book are based on the training, personal experiences, and research of the author. Because each person and situation is unique, the editors and publisher urge the reader to check with a qualified health professional before using any procedure where there is any question as to its appropriateness.

The publisher does not advocate the use of any particular diet and exercise program, but believes the information presented in this book should be available to the public.

Because there is always some risk involved, the author and publisher are not responsible for any adverse effects or consequences resulting from the use of any of the suggestions, preparations, or procedures in this book. Please do not use the book if you are unwilling to assume the risk. Feel free to consult a physician or other qualified health professional. It is a sign of wisdom, not cowardice, to seek a second or third opinion.

Cover design by Martin Hochberg and Rudy Shur
Typeset by ACS Graphics, Fresh Meadows, NY


**Library of Congress Cataloging-in-Publication Data**

Kushi, Michio.
  Michio Kushi on the greater view.

  1. Macrobiotic diet--Addresses, essays, lectures.
2. Diet therapy--Addresses, essays, lectures.
3. Diet--Addresses, essays, lectures. 4. Education--
Addresses, essays, lectures. I. East west journal
(Brookline, Mass. : 1978) II. Title.
RM235.K874 1985     613.2′6     85-22828
ISBN 0-89529-269-6 (pbk.)

Printed in the United States of America

10  9  8  7  6  5  4  3  2  1

# CONTENTS

# PREFACE

This book has been slightly delayed in reaching you. We kept it out of the country as long as we could—a hundred years or so.

There's no Aleutian Earth Mother's statue in San Francisco Bay, facing west, with open arms, saying "Send me your sages, your guides, your tireless teachers who hear our yearning to be free." The Statue of Liberty is in New York harbor, with her back turned to Japan.

San Francisco was a staging area for missionaries, outward bound. Coolies were kept out, sent back. "Stay put," they were told, "We'll get around to your salvation later." And then, thirty years ago, between Hiroshima and Hayakawa, a great Japanese teacher slipped through, disguised as a student. Security screening at Greyhound Bus Terminals was in a primitive state; there were major slip-ups in government surveillance all along the way.

Graffiti scrawls began to appear on walls of Valium shooting galleries, intensive care pavilions, terminal cancer cruise ships: "Listen to Kushi." Samizdat copies began passing from hand to hand. Forgotten gospels and ancient epistles began to reappear in the form of new books, looking strangely like this one which bears his name.

These pages ought properly to have been banned, burned—or at the very least smoked. Unless kept out of the reach of children (and former children) the enormous dream therein could envelop us all.

Turn these pages at your own risk. Chew each paragraph at least fifty times. Relax and enjoy.

—William Dufty

# INTRODUCTION

Michio Kushi is most well-known as a teacher of macrobiotics and as a counselor for the ill. However, these aspects of Kushi's work reflect only one part of his total dedication to creating a new world. The remarkable reputation of Kushi, stemming from the many cases of apparent cancer reversals which have occurred through his counselling, has created an image of macrobiotics primarily as a healing program. However, this type of healing, on the personal level, is most valuable only because through changes in the individual can changes be made on the social level. It is his commitment to social change through personal transformation on the biological and spiritual level that has led Kushi to be the most active proponent and teacher of macrobiotics.

Born in 1926, Michio Kushi experienced firsthand the militarism of pre-war Japan. This was followed by the ravages of World War II, which inspired in him a lasting dedication to the cause of peace. After receiving a degree in International Law from Tokyo University, he came to the United States in 1949 to do graduate studies at Columbia University. Gradually disillusioned by the superficiality of various plans for world government, he began to apply the macrobiotic approach of Georges Ohsawa to the transformation of individuals. He felt this was the only practical basis for a lasting fulfillment of humanity's aspiration toward both social peace and personal freedom.

Over the past thirty-five years he has given thousands of lectures, seminars, and consultations which have helped hundreds of thousands of people regain their vitality and health. Through their renewed outlook on life, these people have established healthy families and contributed actively to social regeneration. Kushi's students and friends have been active in creating the modern natural foods and holistic health movements in North America and Europe. He has continued working in the area of health care and is involved in research programs with medical institutions to further substantiate the value of a macrobiotic diet and lifestyle. In addition, Kushi continues to lecture throughout the world in an effort to further the global development of macrobiotics.

His teaching activities in the Boston area are focused on the Kushi Institute, the Kushi Foundation and the East West Foundation. He was the founder of Erewhon Natural Foods Company and the *East West Journal*. He has written *The Macrobiotic Way, The Book of Do-In, How To See Your Health, The Cancer Prevention Diet,* and *Your Face Never Lies: An Introduction to Oriental Diagnosis.* Kushi has also been an inspiration in the writing of many natural and macrobiotic cookbooks, and has fostered the formation of macrobiotic study and teaching centers throughout the world.

The following chapters have been edited from interviews and articles that have appeared in *East West Journal* over the past ten years. The articles are based either on tape recordings that Kushi dictated for publication or on lectures which were attended by *East West Journal* writers and then transcribed. Sherman Goldman, a previous editor of *East West Journal*, was responsible for the majority of the editing and clarification of these transcripts. Kushi's manner of speaking is vivid, direct, and witty, though still influenced by grammatical patterns from his native language of Japanese. While turning the spoken into the written word, we hope that the overall simplicity and clarity of his spirit comes through.

We want to thank Michio Kushi for his help in clarifying our visions of a new world. We hope that through the messages of this book, you, the reader, will also discover valuable insights and lessons to help in the formulation and realization of your image of a new world.

# I
# HEALTH

# 1

# Cancer's Cause and Cure

I recently spoke with a middle-aged woman who was suffering from breast cancer. Before learning about our dietary approach, she had already undergone an operation and received about ten radiation treatments. She had taken medication, consisting of hormone and vitamin therapy, and chemotherapy was now being considered as well. After all of this, she was still considered a borderline case—the cancer had definitely not been controlled.

This woman's case is not unique. Modern medical science has yet to reach any definite conclusions regarding either the cause or treatment of cancer. In fact, there are more cases of cancer now than when concentrated research began over thirty years ago.

During 1980 over 750,000 Americans will develop cancer, with 2,100 new cases each day. Over 400,000 cancer patients, 1,100 a day, will die. The triumph of modern medicine, which began its development about one hundred years ago, is now reflected in magnificent hospitals, elaborate technologies, and highly trained specialists. But the strength and splendor of all these accomplishments is now being seriously challenged by the problem of cancer.

## THE CONVENTIONAL APPROACH TO CANCER

There are presently two principal theories regarding the cause of cancer. The first is that cancer arises as a result of "cancer-causing substances," including chemicals and preservatives contained in food, chemicals and various pollutants in the environment, such as asbestos or industrial

Originally published in March, 1981 (East West Journal Vol. 11 No. 3)

wastes, and external stimuli such as X-rays or ultra-violet rays. The second major explanation is the "virus theory," arrived at through microscopic examination of cancer cells, revealing the presence of viruses. The presence of virus cells has led to the conclusion that these cells are the cause of the condition, and that cancer might therefore even be infectious.

Other factors are also suspect; for instance, some scientists have begun to think that some defect in the genes passed on to an individual at birth can create a predisposition to cancer later in life, or in other words, that the tendency to develop cancer may be hereditary.

However, none of these theories has resulted in the discovery of a comprehensively effective treatment. The principal discovery to date has been that early detection is the most advisable means of controlling the disease. Furthermore, some of the current diagnostic methods may be contributing to accelerated malignant growth. X-ray scanning for breast or lung tumors, for example, is now commonly suspected of increasing the risk of developing a malignancy in the breast.

Once a cancer is detected, surgical removal of the cancerous tissue or of an entire diseased organ or gland remains the principal method of treatment. Other widely used treatments include medication, radiation therapy, which consists of radioactive bombardment of the cancer cells, and chemotherapy, the injection of powerful chemicals into the bloodstream. There are also various additional forms of treatment currently in the experimental stage, such as thermotherapy or hypothermia (including high fever by subjecting the entire body to intensive heat), immunotherapy (attempting to stimulate the body's native internal defense mechanisms, usually by injections of vitamin A, interferon, or other substances), photoradiation (the injection and laser-excitation of photoactive materials which may transmute into lethal gases, killing the cancerous cells), or Laetrile, the controversial vitamin $B_{17}$, which has recently been legally adopted for experimentation in the United States.

How effective are these treatments? It is difficult to say with certainty, but the evidence so far is not encouraging. For example, authorities have found that childhood cancer victims, treated with radiation and chemotherapy, stand a greater chance than normal children of developing a new cancer in later years. In general, it is estimated that untreated cancer patients actually live up to four times longer than those who receive treatment!

## THE PRESENT CRISIS OF DEGENERATION

When I came to America over thirty years ago, the rate of cancer in this country was approximately one out of fifteen. Today this has jumped to potentially one out of four, or twenty-five percent of the population. If this increase continues at the present rate, 50 percent of the population will develop cancer by the end of this century; and in thirty years from now, virtually everyone will have cancer.

A similar situation exists with other chronic and degenerative disorders. Thirty years ago the rate of mental illness in America was one out of twenty; it has now more than doubled to over one out of ten. Obesity is a recognized risk factor in many of our leading causes of death, including cardiovascular disease, liver disease, diabetes, and others; and obesity, like mental illness, can be severely debilitating even when not fatal. One out of every three Americans is now considered to be overweight to a degree that has significantly reduced their life expectancy.

During the Kennedy administration, millions of dollars were allocated for research on the common cold, yet now, almost twenty years later, there are still no conclusive results. In fact, no major sickness can really be cured by modern methods. In some cases they may be symptomatically controlled, but fundamentally they cannot be cured.

Given these and many other trends, we can clearly see that America, together with our modern civilization as a whole, is now on the verge of self-extinction as a result of deep-seated chronic biological degeneration. The time left to us to reverse this direction is very short. By the time the present generation grows to adulthood, we may be witnessing the complete decline of our recently developed modern way of life; the final collapse may come within the next twenty or at the utmost, forty years.

This failure, however, can also be seen as an opportunity for deep self-reflection. The cancer problem offers the chance to rethink seriously our present understanding of health and sickness and to examine the basic premises of our way of life.

The modern way of thought, for example, usually regards cancer as an aberration caused by certain factors (e.g., virus, genes, or carcinogenic substances) which are viewed as "enemies." To cure the cancer, these "enemies" must be removed, sought out and destroyed, or bombarded by chemicals and radiation. Our modern understanding of life, health, sickness, and the nature of humanity is *dualistic*. Dualistic thinking divides good from bad, friend from enemy, seeing the one as desirable and the other as undesirable. This divisive mode of thought actually underlies all of modern society, including education and religion, politics and economics, science and industry; and it has culminated in the dead end reached by our modern failure to solve the problem of cancer.

As long as our basic point of view is dualistic, it is impossible to fundamentally cure any sickness, whether diabetes, emphysema, leprosy, arthritis, mental illness, or even the common cold. The current mode of attack stems from our ignorance of the true nature of life and health. In a profound sense, while the riddle of cancer is testing our modern medical understanding, it is also challenging modern civilization itself.

## A HOLISTIC VIEW OF CANCER

For the past fifteen years, many people have been seriously studying this larger problem. The first conclusion reached was:

> *If cancer is to be cured, it must first be understood; and if it is to be understood, dualism must be outgrown in favor of a monistic or unified perspective.*

From this perspective we can see that no enemy or conflict really exists. On the contrary, all factors are proceeding in a very harmonious manner, coexisting and supporting each other.

Cancer generally begins as a growth in one specific area, serving the purpose of detoxifying other bodily functions and organs by localizing the body's overall toxic condition. Therefore, while this cancer is developing, the functioning of the other organs and of the body as a whole is able to continue as normal. Cancer is not a disease, then, of certain cells or certain organs. It is a means of self-protection for an entire diseased organism. By removing this cancerous growth, we then allow the toxins to scatter again throughout the body, creating the conditions for another form of sickness or perhaps another localization.

From the perspective of monism, in other words, cancer is seen as an attempt on the part of the body to establish balance. If the cancer is removed, the balance is disrupted and may collapse.

Of primary importance in dealing with cancer is not to disturb this natural mechanism by taking out or destroying the cancer itself. On the contrary, we must totally affirm and approve of the body's natural efforts to maintain a functioning harmony.

Once we cease our efforts to remove the cancer, we are in a position to ask the all-important question, "What has created the toxic condition?" In considering the question, we cannot ignore the pivotal role of our daily food in determining our physiological condition. Over the past fifty years, the types of foods we consume have changed drastically, in composition, quality, processing, and proportion. With the rise of affluence, rich foods such as fatty meats, dairy products, and sugar have become widely available in quantity. Simple, unrefined foods have been overwhelmingly replaced by such items as white bread, orange juice, French fries, cola drinks, processed cheeses and meat products, and a wide range of chemical additives, drugs, and medications.

It is noteworthy that as these foods have become more widely used, the incidences of cancer have risen at a rapidly increasing rate. Any and all of these foods may create a chronically toxic blood condition and therefore be responsible for creating cancer. By positively influencing the physiological quality of our blood cells, lymph, and other body fluids through proper nutrition, we can reverse that toxic quality, and the localization represented by the cancer condition becomes unnecessary. Practically speaking, *potential cancers may be avoided, and existing cancers reversed,* with the correct change in daily food.

If we study traditional eating patterns over the past millennia, we find that the human diet has generally consisted of whole cereal grains, beans, and fresh vegetables, supplemented with seasonal fruits, nuts and seeds, small quantities of lean animal foods, and in some areas edible seaweeds and fermented soybean products. Combined with proper techniques of selection, combination, and cooking, these foods do not produce the chronic toxic condition underlying cancer.

The following standard macrobiotic dietary recommendations have been formulated with universal human dietary traditions in mind and have been further refined over several decades as a result of numerous encounters with cancer and other illnesses. When applied very carefully, they create a stabilized state of overall physiological balance; they may therefore be followed not only for the relief of cancer but also for the correction or prevention of most other disease states as well. This approach may also be safely followed by persons already in generally good health, often with considerable benefits. To heal specific types of cancer, it is necessary to modify the standard diet. Please consult your local East West Center for specific recommendations.

## STANDARD MACROBIOTIC DIETARY APPROACH

1.  At least 50 percent by volume cooked of every meal should be whole cereal grains, prepared by a variety of cooking methods. (Whole cereal grains include brown rice, whole wheat, whole wheat bread, whole wheat chapatis, whole wheat noodles, barley, millet, oats, oatmeal, corn on the cob, corn grits, buckwheat groats [kasha], buckwheat noodles [soba], rye, whole rye bread, etc.) The majority of grain dishes should be in whole form rather than cracked or as flour.

2.  Approximately 25 percent to 35 percent of each meal may include vegetables: two-thirds of them cooked in various styles, including sautéing, steaming, boiling, and baking; up to one-third of them as raw salad. Mayonnaise and all commercial dressings should be avoided. Potatoes, including sweet potatoes and yams, tomatoes, eggplants, asparagus, spinach, beets, zucchini, avocado, and any other vegetables of tropical or semi-tropical origin should be avoided, unless you live in a tropical area.

3.  Approximately 5 percent to 10 percent of daily food intake by volume should include miso soup or natural shoyu broth soup (one or two small bowls daily). The taste should not be too salty. The ingredients should include various vegetables, seaweeds, beans, and grains; alter the recipe often.

4.  From 10 percent to 15 percent of daily intake may include cooked beans and sea vegetables. Beans for daily use are azuki (small red) beans, chick peas, lentils, and black beans. Other beans are for occasional use only. Sea vegetables such as kombu, hijiki, wakame, arame, dulse, nori, agar-agar, and Irish moss can be prepared with a variety of cooking methods. These dishes should be seasoned with a moderate amount of shoyu or sea salt.

5.  Once or twice a week, a small volume of white-meat fish may be easten. The method of cooking should vary each time. Whole small dried fish (iriko) may also be used occasionally as a seasoning. A fruit

dessert, preferably cooked, may also be eaten two or three times a week, provided the fruits grow in the local climatic zone. If you live in a temperate zone, avoid tropical and semi-tropical fruits. Fruit juice is not advisable, except for occasional consumption in very hot weather. Roasted seeds or nuts (with a slight salt taste), dried fruits, or roasted beans may occasionally be enjoyed as snacks or supplements.

6. Beverages recommended include bancha twig tea (kukicha), mu tea, dandelion tea, and cereal grain coffee, all for daily use, as well as any traditional tea that does not have an aromatic fragrance or stimulant effect.

7. Foods to be avoided for the betterment of health include:
   - Meat, animal fat, poultry, dairy food, eggs, all fatty or greasy foods.
   - Tropical or semi-tropical fruits and fruit juices; soft drinks, all commercial, artificial drinks and beverages; coffee, colored tea, and all aromatic stimulant teas such as peppermint, rose hips, etc.
   - Sugar, honey, all syrups, saccharin, and other concentrated or artificial sweeteners. (Rice honey, barley malt, or maple syrup may be used in very small quantities for an occasional sweet taste).
   - All refined, polished grains and flours, and the derivatives of these flours.
   - All chemicalized foods, such as colored, preserved, highly processed, sprayed, or chemically treated foods.
   - All mass-produced, industrialized foods, including canned food and frozen food.
   - Hot spices, any aromatic, stimulant food, food accessories or artificial beverages; artificial vinegar, MSG, or any other commercial seasonings.

8. Additional suggestions:
   - Cooking oil should be of vegetable origin; for maximum health, limit oil to unrefined sesame or corn oil, used only in very moderate volume.
   - Salt should always be white unrefined sea salt. Natural shoyu and miso, prepared in the traditional way, may be used for seasoning in cooking.
   - The following condiments are recommended for use at the table: gomasio (10 to 14 parts roasted sesame seeds to 1 part sea salt); roasted kelp, kombu, or wakame powder; shredded nori, shio

kombu, or boiled nori; umeboshi salt plums; tekka; natural shoyu (moderate use, only for taste).

- You may eat two or three times per day regularly, as much as you want, provided the proportions of different foods are correct and chewing is thorough. Please avoid eating for approximately three hours before sleeping. For thirst, you may drink a small volume of fresh water but not iced.

9.  Final advice: Proper preparation of food is so vitally important that everyone is advised to learn the macrobiotic way of cooking by attending cooking classes given by experienced teachers and by trying out recipes in macrobiotic cookbooks.

# 2

# From Herpes to Hysterectomy

All things in nature can be divided into two: day and night, birth and death, spring and fall, man and woman, sperm and egg. One category is created more by the force of centrifugality or expansion, known in the Orient as "yin." The other, complementary category is created by the force of centripetality or contraction, known as "yang." "Yin" and "yang," although ancient terms, are still used throughout the Orient. And although the terminology may be different, a similar view of nature and universe is common to many cultures in both East and West, North and South.

On earth these forces appear as the forces of heaven and earth. Spiralling in from infinite space, heaven's force—which includes cosmic rays, electromagnetic and light radiation, solar energy, and air pressure—moves in a counterclockwise motion, in the same direction as the rotation of the Earth. In the Orient, this more yang force is called the "energy of heaven." Earth's more yin force is generated outward by the rotation of the planet and spirals clockwise to the periphery of space. (These directions are opposite in the Southern Hemisphere.) In the Orient, it is known as the "energy of earth." Between these two antagonistic, yet complementary motions, all things on the earth and in the relative, ever-changing world are created, maintained, destroyed, and eventually reborn into the eternal cycle of life. Nothing can exist by one force alone; both forces are active in every phenomenon.

Originally published in October, 1983 (East West Journal Vol. 13 No. 10)

## WOMEN AND EARTHLY ENERGY

While men are primarily influenced by heaven's force due to its greater attraction to their male chromosomal charge—earth's force predominates in women. The female reproductive organs develop a more upward and inward structure, while the male sex organs develop in a more outward and downward manner.

As the more powerful earth's force passes through the body of a female in the womb, it meets the force of heaven flowing in the opposite direction. When these forces collide, deep within the intestinal region, they create a pair of spirals which later develop into the Fallopian tubes and ovaries. Since the influence of heaven's force is less, the female develops a clitoris rather than a penis. When a collision occurs in the area of the heart, the resulting spirals of energy eventually take the form of mammary glands and breasts. In men, this collision creates a pair of spirals which become nipples, but not expanded breasts.

Heaven and earth's forces run along an invisible channel located deep within the body. The seven centrally charged regions along this channel of energy were called *chakras* in ancient India. The intensive charge of energy that they produce is distributed throughout the body, activating and giving life to all of its functions.

Thus energy flows from heaven and earth through the human body, but it can become blocked and stagnated. Through extremes of eating, inactivity—both physical and mental—and other material and spiritual factors, tumors and cysts can form, infections can easily arise, menstrual periods can become irregular and painful, and the emotional life suffers. In the following sections, after a closer look at the female reproductive organs, some of the more common manifestations of energy blockage will be examined, as well as natural ways to "unblock the energy."

## THE SEX ORGANS

The female sex organs, taking the shape created by earth's energy, are composed of outer and inner organs. The external organs, or vulva, consist of the labia majora and the labia minora (outer and inner lips)—the folds of soft skin which surround and protect the vagina; and the clitoris, the small erectile organ which becomes filled with blood during sexual activity.

The internal sex organs are the vagina, a muscular tube which extends upward and backward from the vulva; the cervix, the narrow neck of the uterus; the uterus, or womb, a pear-shaped, hollow organ which lies in the center of the lower abdomen; a pair of oviducts, or Fallopian tubes, about five inches long, which extend from the top of the uterus to the ovaries; and the ovaries, almond-shaped glands of reproduction located on either side of the uterus.

The ovaries produce mature egg cells and also hormones. The ovarian hormones play a major role in the changes of the menstrual cycle. In addition, they are responsible for feminine bodily and sexual characteristics. Estrogen especially carries the expansive energy of the earth, through which the female sex organs are created and nourished.

## THE MENSTRUAL CYCLE

### Ovarian Changes

The ovaries are about one and a half inches long and an inch wide. The outer layer of each ovary contains cells each of which produces about 400,000 follicles. The follicle, a spirally formed mass of cells, contains ovum, or egg cell, at its center.

At the beginning of the first menstrual cycle, and at every one that follows, several follicles begin to mature. Usually only one reaches maturity in each cycle while the others degenerate. The menstrual cycle, repeated once every month throughout the reproductive years of a woman's life, begins at the time of menarche, the onset of menstruation, and continues until menopause, the cessation of menstruation.

As a follicle matures it accumulates fluid, increasing in size until it occupies as much as one-fourth of the ovary. The follicle begins to develop when the menstrual period ends. After about ten days, the mature follicle bursts and releases its ovum which then enters the finger-like end of the Fallopian tube. This discharge of the ovum is known as ovulation and occurs about once every twenty-eight days. At this point, lasting from 12 to 24 hours, a woman is fertile. If fertilization occurs, the egg travels to the uterus and embeds itself in the uterine wall; if it does not, the egg travels to the uterus, to be later discharged through menstruation.

**Uterine Changes**

In its contracted state, the uterus, or womb, is about the size of a pear.
Its walls (the myometrium) are one of the strongest muscles in the body.
The uterus expands dramatically during pregnancy.

The internal lining of the uterus, known as the endometrium,
undergoes a series of changes during the menstrual cycle. While the follicle is maturing, cells of the endometrium multiply, causing it to grow
much thicker. Mucus glands grow and new blood vessels develop.

After ovulation, the lining of the uterus becomes even thicker and
glands and blood vessels in it continue to proliferate. The mucus glands
also produce a thick secretion during what is known as the secretory
phase. Then, if fertilization takes place, the endometrium remains in this
condition throughout pregnancy. If it doesn't take place, the upper layers
of the endometrium deteriorate and are discharged through menstruation, along with the ovum.

A woman's menstrual cycle will often correspond to the monthly
phases of the moon, that is, it will follow a regular 28-day cycle.
However, women who eat eggs, meat, dairy products, and sugar often
need more time to discharge excess fat, protein, and water through
menstruation—often five days longer—while women who eat whole
grain and vegetable-based diets usually finish their menstruation within
three days, and accomplish the repair of the endometrium in only one
day.

## COMMON PROBLEMS

Increasingly, in American women, this healthy cycle is disrupted by
organic or hormonal dysfunctions. In addition, infections of the vagina
or urinary tract, and viruses such as herpes, can cause discomfort, pain,
and inconvenience. Following is a look at some of these problems, and
natural ways to eliminate them. The most common reason for their existence is a diet of extremes—eating yin, expansive foods such as sugar,
fruit juice, tropical fruits, milk, stimulants, chemicals, and drugs, as well
as extremely yang, contractive foods—such as meat, eggs, and hard
cheese. When the extremes are eliminated and a balanced diet is followed, and steps are taken to get rid of accumulated toxins, dramatic
results can often be achieved.

## Endometriosis

When a woman develops endometriosis, portions of the endometrium, the lining of the uterus, break away from the uterus and start to grow in other parts of the pelvis, for example, in the Fallopian tubes, ovaries, or on the surface of the bladder or rectum. Endometriosis may or may not produce discomfort in the pelvic region. The most common symptom is pain which begins several days before the start of the menstrual period, most probably caused when the endometrial tissue in various other locations undergoes changes similar to those occuring in the uterine lining.

Endometriosis, which appears to be increasing, is caused by the repeated overconsumption of animal products—fatty, oily foods such as pizza, hamburger, bacon, fried chicken, etc.—as well as sugar, fruits, flour products, stimulants, aromatic foods and beverages, alcohol, drugs and chemicals.

## Infections and Adhesions

Many women with IUDs develop chronic low-grade infections, acute infections, or pelvic abscesses. Pelvic infections also sometimes develop following an abortion. Pelvic adhesions, abnormal weblike conjunctions of adjacent tissues, may occur following the removal of fibroids, ovarian cysts, or tubal pregnancies, or after infections or pelvic surgery.

## Ovarian Cysts and Tumors

When accumulation occurs in and around the ovaries, a variety of cysts and tumors often result. There are dozens of varieties of ovarian growths and each is the result of a specific excessive factor in the diet.

The most common ovarian tumor is the simple cyst which develops when the ovarian follicle does not rupture and release its egg but instead continues growing. These cysts are generally more yin, resulting primarily from the overconsumption of milk, butter, and other light dairy products, sugar, animal fats, and oily and greasy foods.

Another common type of ovarian growth is the dermoid cyst, frequently found in younger women. These may contain hair, fatty material, and calcified matter. Dermoid cysts are more yang, or hard, and arise from the overconsumption of hard, saturated fat such as that in eggs, meat, poultry, and cheese.

### Vaginal Infections

Vaginal infections can come about when foods such as milk, butter, cheese, eggs, chicken, and other animal fats are eaten regularly, or when tropical fruits, sugar, soft drinks, and other extremely yin foods are consumed. Even women who eat a more balanced diet can develop vaginal discharges if too many fruits, nuts, flour products, or oily foods are consumed or if tomatoes, potatoes (especially French fries or potato chips), or white flour products are regularly eaten.

In the most common infection, a thick white discharge is produced. It often comes in clumps and contains yeast or fungus-like organisms known as *monilia*. These infections often cause the labia to become red, swollen, and irritated and may cause pain and burning during urination.

Another common vaginal infection produces a thinner and more yellow-colored discharge which contains a microorganism known as *trichomonas vaginalis*. It often causes an itching sensation which seems to be centered inside the vagina.

Other common infections include a clear thin discharge which results from excessive mucus in the cervix and vaginal wall and a green discharge which may contain pus as a result of an acute infection.

Clear discharges are generally the least serious, while white discharges often preceded the development of a softer type of cyst. Yellowish discharges frequently accompany cysts, while greenish discharges—particularly those that are chronic—may indicate a tendency to develop cancer of the reproductive organs.

### Fibroids

Fibroids are fleshy growths within or on the wall of the uterus. They consist of masses of fibrous tissue and may be single or multiple, large or small. They often resemble a group of marbles.

Fibroids are widespread among women today. They are the result of an extreme diet, especially one containing the heavy saturated fat of meat, dairy, and poultry in combination with extremely yin foods such as sugar, tropical fruits, oil, soft drinks, and refined flour products. When these foods are eaten regularly, mucus and fat begin to build up in the body. This buildup begins at first in areas of the body which connect to the outside, such as the sinuses, breasts, lungs, intestines, kidneys and ovaries, uterus and Fallopian tubes.

The deposits of mucus and fat that build up around the ovaries and uterus often solidify into cysts and tumors. When solidification occurs in the muscle of the uterus, the result is a fibroid tumor. Fibroids often begin as small seedlings. Whether or not they enlarge depends on the quality and volume of excess that is deposited in the uterine region. Frequently they continue to grow and begin to bulge either through the outer lining of the uterus or through the endometrium. In some cases, they bulge so far that they are pushed out on a stalk.

Fibroids may or may not produce noticeable symptoms. Symptoms commonly occur between the ages of thirty-five and forty-five, although women of all ages can experience them. One symptom is bleeding, especially in the form of heavy or prolonged periods. Fibroids frequently distort the uterus so that the surface area of the endometrium is increased. A greater amount of endometrial lining is thus produced each month, thereby increasing the menstrual flow. Their fibrous nature also makes it difficult for bleeding to stop. Fibroids may become quite large and begin to cause pain as a result of pressing on organs such as the bladder or rectum.

### Urinary Tract Infections

In many cases, a urinary tract infection starts as cystitis, or bladder infection, and goes on to pyelitis, or infection of the kidney duct, and then to pyelonephritis, or infection of the kidney.

The symptoms of urinary tract infection include pain and burning during urination. A desire to urinate frequently brings meager results. There is pain in the back and, when the kidneys become infected, chills and fever. With mild infections, the temperature often reaches 102 degrees F, but it may rise as high as 104 degrees F in severe cases. The patient may also vomit and feel generally ill. In severe cases, mucus and blood are present in the urine.

These infections generally come about when the condition of the person has been weakened through more yin foods and drinks.

### HERPES SIMPLEX INFECTION

Every year, an estimated ten million people in the United States develop some form of a sexually contracted disease. In the past, the term "venereal disease" was used to describe these disorders, the major ones being syphilis and gonorrhea. More recently, however, over twenty different diseases that can be spread through sexual contact have been identified. Society is now in the midst of an epidemic of these disorders, and information about them has become increasingly complex.

To illustrate the macrobiotic approach to sexually transmitted diseases (STD), let us consider the example of genital herpes, a problem which now affects increasing numbers of people.

Herpes simplex, the virus of genital herpes, comes in two types: herpes symplex virus type 1 (HSV-1) and herpes simplex virus type 2 (HSV-2). Type 1 is generally more yin and mostly affects the upper regions of the body, especially the head and neck. Its symptoms are clusters of small red lumps around the lips that turn into painful blisters, often referred to as cold sores or fever blisters. The most yang type 2 virus affects the lower regions of the body and is associated with painful lesions around the genitals, buttocks, and thighs. Both varieties can be transmitted through sexual contact. Not all genital herpes is the result of a type 2 infection; an estimated 25 percent of genital infections are the result of the type 1 virus.

Unlike other forms of STD, herpes does not respond to antibiotics. At present it is considered an incurable illness. Among women who are infected with the type 2 virus for the first time, many show no noticeable symptoms. Among those who do have symptoms, small fluid-filled blisters develop on the external sex organs. The blisters are painful and appear within three to twenty days after contact with the virus. If they are located only in the vagina or on the cervix, they may go unnoticed. The blisters soon rupture and the external ones develop into soft open sores that are very painful. The lymph glands in the groin may also become swollen and painful.

An initial outbreak usually lasts about twelve days, after which the illness enters a latent stage. In some cases, the virus remains latent and no additional outbreaks occur. In other cases, it reactivates and the symptoms return, as often as twice a month or as rarely as once every ten years. Recurrences are generally less severe than the initial outbreak. An outbreak of genital herpes of either type can have very severe consequences during pregnancy and childbirth.

The macrobiotic approach to herpes is based on at least reducing, and preferably avoiding, foods which weaken the immune system and provide a fertile ground for the virus to take root, while at the same time eating foods which strengthen the body's natural defenses.

The time needed for recovery depends on a number of factors—particularly on the severity of the condition. Lighter or more recently acquired cases can be healed completely in as little as three weeks, while longer or more severe cases may take up to six months. During this time, keep the skin of the affected area clean and dry.

## DIETARY RECOMMENDATIONS

In order to treat and prevent these conditions, it is important to avoid the extreme foods that caused them to develop. The following dietary suggestions can, in most cases, be applied for the treatment of fibroids, endometriosis, infections and adhesions, ovarian cysts (with slight variations for each type), and vaginal infections. Urinary tract infections and herpes simplex also require slight adjustments. These are guidelines only and not detailed descriptions. For example, for some conditions a small amount of oil may be used, while for others it is best to completely avoid it. It is urged that a person embarking on this course of treatment see a qualified macrobiotic counselor for a diet specifically tailored to her needs, and take macrobiotic cooking classes from an experienced cook.

The standard macrobiotic diet of whole grains, beans, fresh local vegetables, seaweeds, and miso soup, prepared according to macrobiotic principles, can serve as the basis for the recovery process. It is best to minimize flour products, as these can cause mucus, even if whole grain flours are used. It is advisable to use oil only a few times a week; a small amount of good quality sesame or corn oil can then be used to make sautéed vegetables or fried rice. Hard leafy greens such as kale, collards, watercress, and turnip and daikon greens, can be eaten every day. Cooked daikon, daikon greens and kombu, or shredded daikon cooked with kombu and tamari are two dishes that are also good for these conditions; they can be eaten several times a week. Generally, it is better to have a boiled rather than a raw salad, and to use azukis, chick peas, lentils, and black soybeans rather than other kinds of beans. Tempeh and tofu may be eaten a few times a week.

Sea vegetables are important, since minerals are needed for the smooth discharge of toxins from the body. Besides cooking them in soups or with beans or vegetables, they may be eaten in small side dishes a few times a week or made into seaweed condiments.

During the healing process fruit is limited to a small amount of cooked or dried, temperate-climate varieties; avoid raw fruit and fruit juice. Squash, cabbage, daikon, and other sweet-tasting vegetables can be eaten instead of sweets. Nuts and nut butters are best avoided as they contain large amounts of oil and fat. It is also better not to eat animal foods, but if it is strongly desired, to eat only a small serving of white-meat fish.

## EXTERNAL APPLICATIONS

The following external applications are helpful in dissolving fibroid tumors and ovarian cysts and tumors. The hip bath and douche can also be taken for vaginal infections and are also helpful for treating endometriosis.

### The Ginger Compress Followed by the Taro Potato Plaster

These external remedies can be applied to the lower abdomen every day for a period of ten to fourteen days. However, don't apply the ginger compress for more than five minutes and don't apply it without following a taro potato plaster. The ginger compress is here used to prepare the body for the taro plaster.

To prepare the ginger compress, grate a golf-ball-size piece of fresh ginger and place it in a square of cheesecloth. Tie up the ends. Bring a pot of water to just below the boiling point. Squeeze the ginger into the pot, then lower the sack into the pot. Do not boil the ginger, but keep the water just below the boiling point. Dip a towel into the ginger water, wring it out tightly, and apply, as hot as possible, to the area to be treated. A second, dry towel can be placed on top to hold in the heat. If the first towel becomes cool before five minutes, put another hot towel in its place.

To prepare the taro plaster, pare the skin from the potato and grate the white interior. Mix with five percent grated fresh ginger. Spread this mixture, half-an-inch thick, onto a piece of clean cotton linen. Apply with the taro side directly on the skin. Leave it on for three or four hours, or overnight. If the plaster burns, omit the grated ginger. The ginger–taro application may be used once a day for a ten- to fourteen-day period, during which time it is important to eat very strictly. Following this initial period, the ginger–taro application can be used several times a week for an additional six weeks.

Taro potato, also known as *albi*, is available in most North American cities, often in Chinese, Armenian, or Puerto Rican grocery stores or in natural foods stores. Smaller potatoes are the most effective for the plaster. If taro isn't available, a plaster using regular potatoes may be substituted. While not as effective as taro in collecting stagnated toxic matter and drawing it out of the body, it will still produce a beneficial result. Mix 50 to 60 percent grated potato with 40 to 50 percent crushed green leafy vegetables. Crush the ingredients together in a suribachi and apply as above, following the ginger compress.

## HIP BATH

A hot hip bath is a very effective remedy for a variety of disorders. The bath water should contain dried leafy vegetables such as daikon or turnip greens. To prepare them, hang fresh leaves out of direct sunlight. Leave them until they turn brown and brittle. Place four or five bunches of dried leaves in a large pot. If leafy greens aren't available, use two handfuls of arame seaweed instead. Add four to five quarts of water and bring to a boil. Reduce the flame to medium and boil until the water turns brown. Add a handful of sea salt and stir well to dissolve.

Run hot water in the bathtub and add the mixture together with another large handful of sea salt. Fill the tub with just enough water to cover the body from the waist down. Sit in the tub and cover the upper body with a thick cotton towel to prevent chills and absorb perspiration. If the water begins to cool, add more hot water. Stay in the bath for ten to twelve minutes.

The hot bath will cause the lower body to become very red as circulation is increased. The bath also causes a loosening of fat and mucus deposits in the pelvic regions.

### Douche

A special douching solution can be used immediately after the hip bath. To prepare it, either squeeze the juice from half a lemon or add one or two teaspoons of rice vinegar to warm bancha tea. Add a three-finger pinch of sea salt, and stir. This douching solution helps to dislodge deposits of mucus and fat which have been loosened during the hip bath. The hip bath and douch can be repeated every day for up to ten days. During this time, it is important to eat very well and to completely avoid the foods which have contributed to the problem.

# 3

# Reorienting the Male Spirit

Humanity's primary orientation, like that of all biological life, is the survival and development of the species. However, in modern times we are trying to do this strictly through material gain and material power—beyond what is necessary for survival and development. In other words, men are using their traditional role as provider and protector for excessive mastery over nature and the creation of a societal structure far beyond natural needs. With this orientation men have created the class systems, educational systems, political systems, medical systems, and engineering and technological systems. And men have built the wars as well.

Until the beginning of the Industrial Revolution women generally were not as involved in the building of these institutions. Since that time, however, women have begun to compete with men for position and power. The central biological position of women as nourisher and keeper of the species has begun to collapse, and both women and men have become dissatisfied. Men subconsciously miss the supportive, emotional center women used to provide. So men have become frustrated, depressed, and anxious, without understanding why. More and more, men are becoming some kind of psychological monster; it has become necessary to explain what a man is, and what he should be.

Men try to justify their existence through material gain, through technology, but this is a delusion. Because of this delusion humanity is suffering disorder and disease. Society is degenerating into war, monetary struggle, power politics, betrayal, cheating, lies, fear, anx-

---

Originally published in February, 1984 (East West Journal Vol. 14 No. 2)

ieties, and all sorts of crime. Men are having to constantly struggle, and are losing wife and children and home.

Modern medicine with its radiation, chemotherapy, genetic engineering, and the like, is bringing about the rise of an artificial species. Through the disappearance of natural qualities comes a distortion of the species—even though we maintain our form as human beings, we have become almost non-humans. This new, weakened species will collapse very easily before the middle of the next century, even if we don't have World War III. This is the biggest problem humanity is facing.

A sign of this degenerating and degradation is the extent to which men are losing their male qualities. Impotence and infertility are vastly higher today than even fifty years ago. Prostate problems, weak or no sperm, high blood pressure—all combine with the epidemic of women's reproductive problems (hysterectomies, ovarian cysts, chaotic menstruation) to cause the diminishing of the natural human species.

Most of this degeneration can be blamed both on poor eating habits and on psychological conditions. Too much animal food, refined sugar, and artificial chemicals combine with frustration, depression, arrogance, anger, and insecurity, and social, environmental, and working stress, to undermine the health of the species.

And now, in the case of AIDS, diet has become even more chaotic and unbalanced, with overconsumption of more yin, expansive foods and chemicals. People are eating more dairy, more sugar, and tropical fruits such as bananas every day, in addition to soft drinks, and very oily, greasy foods. They are eating less vegetables and whole grains, and even less of the standard American foods such as meats and fish in order to make some kind of balance. This way of eating tends to make people prefer artistic or intellectual pursuits out of balance with physical ones. Physiologically, it disrupts and dissolves the body's immune system and causes what we call AIDS. The resulting lack of physical strength, energy, and immunity to disease, can be expressed as a loss of the power of survival, a loss of the sustaining power of the human species.

So, the question is how to recover natural immunity and natural survival ability, and how to turn around the degeneration of the human species. Modern medicine is not the answer; its approach only advances our unnatural status.

We must use, then, the natural way to recover and build up our original biological strength. That means we do not use chemically synthesized food, but rather organic, natural-quality, naturally-processed whole foods. In order to maintain our human integrity we should use traditional human food, such as whole grains, vegetables, and beans, along with sea salt and seaweeds to maintain our natural evolutionary process. We should reduce as much as possible all unnatural factors such as tropical fruits in a temperate zone, canned, frozen or radioactively treated foods, and various artificial non-foods.

Along with the change to a wholesome diet, men must become physically active. We should take time and discipline ourselves to exercise so that natural energy can flow and be released. Some kind of exercise—running, playing tennis, chopping wood—is necessary. Make sure to walk up stairs instead of taking the elevator, and walk to work instead of driving.

Gradually, as lifestyle changes, natural immune power—natural sustaining strength—will come back. This is the only way the human species, man and woman alike, can be secure.

# 4

# Marijuana—Withdrawal from Wonderland

Over the past fifteen years I have given dietary recommendations to thousands of young people who wanted to stop using marijuana and similar drugs. In fact the drug culture and the macrobiotic movement began to gain prominence in America around the same time, toward the middle and especially the end of the 1960s. Because of that coincidence, many people had the false impression that these two phenomena were similar or identical, whereas in fact they are quite opposite. The confusion was further increased by the fact that some of the young leaders in macrobiotics at that time had formerly been smugglers and well-known drug dealers in San Francisco, Los Angeles, and New York.

As I came to know these people better, I noticed that they seemed to share in common a peculiar kind of difficulty in following a macrobiotic diet. When I understood their problem, I advised the macrobiotic study houses where they were living to making particular allowance for this factor. In general, people who had formerly used large amounts of marijuana and similar drugs on a regular basis all seemed to practice the macrobiotic way of eating in a very rigid, narrow, and almost fanatical manner. They expected that such an extreme approach would lead to immediate and fantastic results, including a kind of higher consciousness. I saw that we had to emphasize a much more relaxed, common-sense application of macrobiotic dietary principles in order to balance their excessively conceptual approach. The young people in question seemed to consider brown rice as some sort of instant solution, in the same way they had formerly looked upon drugs. In reality, the macrobiotic way of life is nothing but a common-sense tradition that involves a great deal of pa-

Originally published in March, 1979 (East West Journal Vol. 9 No. 3)

tience and flexibility in allowing for variations between individual con-
stitutions, climactic factors, and social considerations. Rather than promoting one simplistic answer, it is oriented toward developing our innate
powers of judgment so that we can welcome every difficulty as an opportunity for development. It seemed very difficult for people coming to
macrobiotics from the drug culture to grasp the scope and breadth of the
macrobiotic approach.

As I talked with them about their previous experiences and education,
I saw that they had basically two kinds of reasons for using drugs. In the
first place, many were looking for a new kind of mental or spiritual insight from drugs after they had been very concerned about, then disillusioned by, the current state of our civilization. The second major reason
for smoking marijuana was a need for relaxation from mental and
physical tension.

I sympathize with these very natural and understandable desires, but
at the same time I would recommend a sounder way to reach these goals,
which can also have a deep and enduring effect on society at large. A
sense of meaning as well as a more relaxed approach to life can be gained
in the most reasonable way by developing ways of life that include increasing freedom from the artificial substances, methods of working, and
types of thinking that characterize today's "quick results" civilization.
That instant kind of approach generally has undesirable side-effects in
the long run and is not found in more traditional societies. America is
thus the subject of jokes and anecdotes around the world that play off the
"express" orientation of TV dinners, vending machines, microwave
cooking, instant coffee and so on. Ironically, the young people who use
marijuana and similar substances usually say they prefer natural or
traditional over artificial or modern ways, yet they continue to use drugs,
which belong to this recent category of instant methods.

Fortunately, over the years I have been able to see many thousands of
people in America, Europe, South America, and the Far East recovering
their physical, mental, and spiritual vitality and establishing a clear sense
of brotherhood and sisterhood with all humanity by eliminating the artificial elements in their lifestyle and diet, including hallucinogens, and
returning to a more sound, common-sense orientation. Many of them
have told me stories about their former drug taking, and their experiences exhibit the same general pattern. The immediate results of sudden relaxation and a feeling of expanded consciousness are followed in
the long run by growing fatigue, mental fogginess, and an inability to

react with sufficient quickness to confront the normal challenges of daily life.

On common-sense grounds alone, this sequence is understandable as the inevitable working of the dynamic balance that underlies physiological, psychological, and all other natural phenomena. Prolonged intake of substances which have such dramatically expanding effects must eventually weaken the nervous and other major systems of the body. More specifically, the signs of this process appear in seven main areas:

1. *Dulling of the Autonomic Nervous Function.* Initially, marijuana activates both the parasympathetic and the orthosympathetic nervous systems. However, continual extreme stimulation of this sort tends to leave the parasympathetic system less sensitive, with a resulting loss of quickness and accuracy in adapting to the physical environment. As motor coordination is impaired, accidents become more frequent.

2. *Declining Sensitivity.* The sudden increase of sensitivity that smokers of marijuana experience results from its chemical ability to expand cells which have grown abnormally hard and rigid from the heavy consumption of animal fats that characterizes the contemporary American diet. However, prolonged repetition of this expansive action in itself leads to another form of insensitivity, as the cells of the nervous system become semipermanently expanded and thus lose their natural reactive powers.

3. *Loss of Clarity.* Marijuana affects the inner area of the brain, especially the midbrain, rather than the surrounding cerebral cortex. In its anatomical structure, as well as in the circuits of electromagnetic current which flow through it carrying information, the brain consists of several orbits arranged in a continuous spiral. The midbrain, which is located at the central terminus of these orbits, may be compared to a computer gathering information from the entire nervous system in the form of stimuli; it then relays information outward to appropriate parts of the body in the form of various responses such as speech, decisions to act, etc. In order for this key function to operate well, the innermost orbit of the nervous system, which is situated at the midbrain, must be tightly coiled and highly energized, with its cells compact. The habitual expansion produced by the chemical action of marijuana and similar "mind expanding" drugs has a damaging ef-

fect on mental clarity after a period of time, although the initial impression may be one of relaxation and heightened clarity.

4. *Weakening of Internal Organs.* In terms of yin (expansion) and yang (contraction), certain of our internal organs rely primarily on contraction for their normal activity and others depend more on relaxation. Like the midbrain, whose functioning is impaired by the expansive tendency of marijuana, the major relatively yang organs tend to be weakened by marijuana and similar drugs. They include the spleen, pancreas, heart, lungs, liver and kidneys. Which of these are affected to a noticeable extent depends on a number of individual considerations, including constitution, previous illnesses, former diet, and so on.

5. *Decline in Sexual Vitality.* At first marijuana may heighten sexual sensitivity; however, its continued use creates imbalances in the quantity and quality of hormonal secretions, such as testosterone, from abnormal stimulation of the adrenal, gonadal, and pituitary glands. This imbalance in the hormone system, when combined with general weakening of the nervous system, leads to debility and irregular functioning of the reproductive system.

6. *Degeneration of Red Blood Cell Quality.* Marijuana and similar drugs tend to destroy the intestinal flora which are essential for smooth absorption of food into the blood stream. The liver, spleen, and bone marrow, involved in the continued regeneration of red blood cells, are adversely affected by prolonged use of marijuana. Therefore, people who already suffer from mild forms of illnesses associated with lowered blood quality—such as leukemia, diabetes, asthma, and various skin diseases—tend to experience a worsening of their condition after prolonged marijuana use.

7. *Psychological and Social Impairment.* These various manifestations of lessened physical and mental vitality combine to impede the individual and social development of people burdened with them. They are increasingly unable to strive for the realization of their ideals, or life dreams, and start to prefer only the more sensory, sentimental, and temporary pleasures or comforts. They become less able to renew and maintain their solidarity with others in relationships that require long-term commitments, such as communication with parents or various forms of common intellectual endeavors.

The burgeoning intake of yin (expansive) sustances such as marijuana, LSD, and cocaine—as well as many legal drugs, including amphetamines, tranquilizers, and numerous other medications—is understandable as a natural response to the accelerating consumption of animal products in the form of meat and especially dairy food, such as eggs and cheese, all of which have a generally yang (contractive) effect on our physiology. The current unparalleled use of drugs in America is an unconscious attempt to make balance for the equally unprecedented dietary pattern of modern civilization which, over the past fifty years, has substituted meat and dairy for whole grains as the staple food. Instead of oatmeal porridge, corn muffins, buckwheat pancakes, whole wheat bread or similar traditional forms of cereal grain, a typical modern breakfast, for example, often consists of ham or bacon and two or even three eggs, with the other daily meals correspondingly high in animal food. Animal food can be useful on rare occasions for certain forms of concentrated physical labor, especially in a northern climate with very cold weather; however on a daily basis it is excessive in our temperate climate for the sedentary activity that most Americans engage in. Therefore the breakfast bacon and eggs must be balanced by extremely yin items such as coffee, orange juice from the tropics, and refined, chemicalized cereals highly flavored with white sugar.

The rise in consumption of sugar, citrus fruit, and soft drinks is in fact complementary to our steadily increasing intake of animal products. As animal food forms a larger and larger part of our modern diet—with spectacular recent rises in the use of milk products, particularly cheese—the yin factors in sugar, fruit juices, and even alcohol become inadequate to balance this overwhelming accumulation of yang intake, and the only substances powerful enough to compensate are the increasingly popular drugs, whether illicit or prescription.

Countries which do not consume animal products to the extent that characterizes America's present way of eating also are free of serious drug problems. In fact, foreigners coming from those parts of the world have a spontaneous adverse reaction to marijuana, with symptoms of dizziness, vomiting, heart palpitation, and feelings of panic. Furthermore, Americans who have changed their diet from the prevalent modern one to a more traditional macrobiotic way and who formerly felt the need to smoke marijuana or use similar drugs gradually lose these extreme desires. This natural disappearance of interest in drugs does not occur among so-called New Age lacto-vegetarians or ovo-vegetarians, since their intake of dairy food perpetuates the need for extremely strong yin, not only in the form of honey and supplements such as vitamin C pills, but also in the occasional use of marijuana.

Just as consumption of sugar, alcoholic beverages, and finally drugs is complementary to the rising intake of animal products, the modern superstition that we should take vitamin supplements is a response to the recent practice of refining foods to the point where they are deprived of many vitamins, minerals, and other essential factors. This pattern of interfering unnecessarily with nature—and then turning to even more artificial practices in an attempt to remedy the damage—typifies the wastefulness of modern approaches; it ignores the complementarity that unifies all natural phenomena into organic wholes. By attempting to bypass that basic, common-sense principle of balance, we continually endanger the environment, the economy, and our own health.

The latest swing from one compensatory extreme to the other is the fad of ginseng among users of marijuana and vitamin supplements. The popular notion that ginseng is a healthful product which Oriental people took regularly for vitality and longevity is completely false. Actually only a minute percentage of people in the Far East used ginseng, and even then only once or twice in their lives as an emergency medication.

I would advise against the current practice of using ginseng on an almost daily basis, since it can result in constriction of the heart, with serious effects on the circulatory system. Ginseng is an extremely yang (contractive) substance, because it is the root of a very cold-resistant plant that grows in northern climates; in this sense it is at the extreme pole of complementarity from marijuana, which contains very yin (expansive) factors due to its origin in the leaves of a fast-growing tropical plant. Root and leaf, alkaline and acid, slow and fast rates of growth, northern and southern origin, all offer clues to the yang (contractive) and yin (expansive) tendencies which complement each other in nature as a whole. Intuitively aware of this balancing principle, traditional doctors would give ginseng for an overly yin condition and marijuana for an excessively yang condition on very rare occasions.

People who have been weakened by continual use of extremely yin substances such as marijuana are understandably prone to accept the myth that the ginseng they naturally feel attracted to was part of daily life in the Orient. Equally mistaken is the popular notion that native peoples in tropical countries such as India, Peru, and central parts of Africa used marijuana or similar substances on a regular daily basis. In fact, only a few tribes used marijuana, and, when they did, it was only as a medication or on rare ceremonial occasions. The popularity of myths about the regular use of marijuana and hallucinogens among native citizens is understandable: it merely reflects the irresistible craving people feel for extreme relaxants after they have consumed animal products in excess over a period of many years. The attraction between yin and yang is as inevitable as our desire to drink liquids after we have eaten very salty food; therefore it is not a phenomenon to be judged moralistically or criminalized by legislation.

Since the increasing use of marijuana and other expansive drugs, both illicit and prescription, is a biological phenomenon, I do not favor the approach which tries to control that pattern through legal punishments or moral persuasion. Such efforts are bound to be useless since they ignore the underlying cause, which is physiological. At different times in modern history, attempts have been made to outlaw on moral grounds various types of behavior whose real cause is biological—practices such as homosexual activity, drinking alcohol, performing abortions, etc. All such laws prove impossible to enforce, because wherever artificial impositions appear in human society, because wherever artificial impositions appear in human society, they inevitably evoke widespread opposition. Part of our human dignity involves learning through experience and observation how to take responsibility for our own lives, including our health as individuals. Each family also is responsible for the health and happiness of its members. The appearance of laws such as prohibition of alcohol consumption or criminalization of marijuana smoking in modern society is a sign that education has been defective in the place where it naturally starts, the home. In order to reverse the present trend toward increasing drug use, the following three methods are available:

1. Education on the effects of drug use can be emphasized through public media, government information offices, religious organizations, schools, and, most important, the home. This approach would be effective in many cases, especially if developed in the setting of a family where the parents can serve as examples for living in a healthy way.
2. Society can leave the decision on marijuana use up to the discretion of each individual. In this way, some people will discover from their

own experience that marijuana smoking is harmful to their health and will give it up; others will not try it, because they can observe its unhealthy effects on those who use it; a third class will use it and, unable to realize that it is causing a decline in their health, will continue to the point of completely losing their ability to cope with daily life. This method is the one actually being used at present, as laws prove to be unenforceable. It has the advantage of letting all people exercise their freedom and take responsibility for their destiny, although it has the disadvantage that some end miserably.

3. The third approach, which I would recommend, is a biological one, eliminating the need for marijuana and other drugs by substantially reducing the present levels of animal food consumption. A widespread change in dietary patterns along these lines would, of course, have major repercussions on our economy. However, such a direction has already been suggested by the Senate Select Subcommittee on Nutrition and Human Needs in its 1977 report, "Dietary Goals," in the context of reducing various chronic diseases, and the potential economic dislocations could be provided for by careful long-term planning.


This third, physiological method also involves some psychological pitfalls, however, which should be clarified. In my observation, many people who formerly took large amounts of drugs develop an overwhelming craving for whole grains once they begin to eat these traditional foods. They seem to have a very strong sensation that they have finally discovered the truly nourishing food which they had actually been searching for in vain during their years of mental and physical confusion while taking drugs. Therefore, they have a sometimes dangerous tendency to limit their diet within extremely narrow bounds. Regardless of its alarming effects on their physical and mental vitality, they will follow a very rigid diet for a long period of time, eating 80 percent, 90 percent, or even 100 percent whole grains (brown rice, buckwheat, millet, barley, rye, corn, whole wheat, etc.) with very little or no vegetables or other types of foods. Since their excretory, digestive, and nervous systems have been damaged through their former abuse of drugs, they tend to develop the following serious symptoms while adhering to such a narrow diet: anemia, extreme loss of weight, low vitality, a psychological tendency to be overly conceptual in their manner of thinking, stubbornness, narrow-mindedness and exclusivity to a degree bordering on fanaticism.

Therefore I would recommend that anyone who has taken many drugs in the past and who wishes to change his or her diet toward a more traditional orientation do so in a very gradual and moderate way. Specifically I would suggest the following guidelines:

1. Whole grains should account for 40 to 60 percent of food intake by cooked volume and should be prepared in a variety of styles—casseroles, breads, pancakes, noodles, porridge, muffins, crackers, etc.

2. Vegetables should account for 20 percent to 30 percent of food intake, cooked in a variety of styles, with a small portion served raw in the form of salads and pickles.

3. Beans should account for approximately 10 percent of the intake, cooked in a variety of styles, including traditional fermented soy products such as tempeh, miso, and soy sauce, to further the reestablishment and normal growth of beneficial intestinal flora.

4. Cooked sea vegetables should account for approximately 5 percent of intake. Because of their high mineral content they are particularly useful in restoring those parts of the nervous system damaged by drugs.

5. Fish and seafood, fruit, nuts and seeds should account for roughly another 5 percent of intake, varying with individual needs and time of year—e.g., more fruit in summer than in winter, and a dinner of fish as often as once or even twice a week in winter. This fifth class of foods is particularly recommended for older people.

6. Liquids may be consumed as freely as desired, although stimulants such as coffee and alcoholic beverages should be minimized.

7. All food should be chewed very well, and some form of sensible physical exercise should be practiced every day.

These general suggestions, if followed in a common-sense manner with minor variations upon occasion, will lead to restoration of the damage done by drug abuse and will not produce any serious reactions. The effects of taking marijuana and similar potent drugs do not, however, disappear overnight. In my observation, the following timetable generally applies:

| DURATION OF SMOKING MARIJUANA ONCE A WEEK OR MORE | PERIOD TO RECOVER FROM THE EFFECTS |
|---|---|
| 1–4 weeks | 4 months |
| 1–3 months | 1 year |
| 4–6 months | 2 years |
| 6 months–1 year | 3 years |
| 1–2 years | 4–5 years |
| 3–5 years | 6–7 years |

Until the period of recovery is complete, all of the foods listed in the suggested guidelines should be included on a regular basis, *with the percentage of grains not rising much above 60 percent* (or falling below 40 percent) for any considerable length of time. Other foods may be increased according to personal desires—e.g., sea vegetables may be 10 percent instead of 5 percent, or beans may be 15 percent instead of 10 percent. After the recovery period is over, the percentage of grains may, of course, be increased, with very beneficial results—but not until then.

The common mistake of former drug users who adopt a macrobiotic diet is to seek quick results by eating a very high percentage of grains. The body may then begin to eliminate its stored toxins through the skin, since the urinary system has not yet regained its full functioning. These abnormal discharges of mucus or pus appear in the form of boils or small tumor-like growths usually on the extremities, particularly the legs and hands. These painful discharges will sometimes dry up and disappear in a short time, but when they appear in several places at the same time, they may become infected, developing serious inflammation. Here, at the very first appearance of such discharges, the percentage of vegetables, fruits and/or fish should be increased and the percentage of grains *decreased* in order to slow down the rate of toxin elimination.

During the period of recovery from drug use, improvement is gradual but may be interrupted by the transitory, occasional reappearance of symptoms associated with the former period when the individual was taking drugs. These minor relapses include the following: occasional experience of a strange or disturbing dream at night, uncanny or weird visual and auditory impressions, unaccountably poor judgment or inaccurate decisions, overexcitement or depression, hyper-sensitivity, general anxiety or feelings of cowardice, laziness or sloppiness, irregularity in writing or speaking, chaotic expression, lack of responsibility and laxness in human relationships, frequent changes of mind and difficulty thinking clearly, fatigue, low resistance to cold weather or infection, slow rate of wound healing, loss of sexual appetite or ability, stiffness, problems with balance, and others.

Which of these symptoms will appear depends on the former medical history of each individual, but none is cause for serious concern, since they generally disappear of themselves as the healing process proceeds. However, one rather serious psychological problem tends to afflict a large percentage of people who have formerly taken drugs to any large extent. Until the period of recovery has been completed, people who have taken drugs have a tendency to wander about aimlessly from one spiritual practice to another, one group of friends to a new set, one job to the next in a continual, erratic shifting of allegiance.

This flightiness, ultimately caused by a general decline in our native powers of judgment, often is manifested as an extreme gullibility toward some of the more shallow religious, psychological, and technological belief systems that abound in modern society. Debility of the central nervous system, at the root of this problem, is caused not only by marijuana smoking, of course, but by the overall intake of strong chemicals, such as medications, which pervade modern life. Faced with the modern onslaught of crises, the growing proportion of the population whose powers of judgment have been weakened through the effects of drug use shuffle endlessly from doctor to doctor, guru to guru, expert to expert, seminar to seminar, and never think of thinking for themselves at all.

Fortunately this shopping mentality can give way to a more grounded intelligence—with a natural immunity to shallow proposals that hold out the promise of miraculous results in record time—as the intuitive power of the nervous system is gradually restored through following a more traditional diet and lifestyle. Although the general decline of public health is accelerating, there is, at the same time, an opposite trend now gathering momentum; it comprises a steadily growing number of people throughout the country who are reorienting their lives in the direction of a sound and traditional yet dynamic balance. The development of this general movement depends on our deepening appreciation and understanding of the Unifying Principle, which creates the natural order in all phenomena through the fundamental law of balance.

Viewed in those terms, even the present degeneration of society can be seen as the reverse side to an emerging movement toward the full recovery of our health, freedom, and happiness. The purpose of that biological revolution is the complete restoration of everyone's native, intuitive, and essentially human strengths. These include a sense of wonder at all phenomena in this perpetually changing universe, trust in each other and capacity for friendship, genuine creativity and inventiveness, keen sensitivity to the beauty of nature, gratitude for our physical and spiritual ancestors, and an endless aspiration. That invincible aspiration, like the phoenix, can never die. It continually emerges from its ashes, for it is one with the law of change, the only constant in this relative world. Through the constant alternation of balanced opposites, everything spirals both inward and outward in a geometric orderliness that grows endlessly toward greater harmony.

# 5

# Heal Thyself

*In a March, 1983 conversation with the* East West Journal, *Michio Kushi discussed his work with cancer patients. As this in-depth interview reveals, Michio Kushi's knowledge of both Eastern spiritual practices and Western science has given him a unique insight into cancer. His advice has been sought by scores of people whose cases were termed "hopeless" by conventional medicine.*

*The* East West Journal *interview is reprinted in its entirety on the pages that follow. The interviewer's questions appear in boldface type, and Michio Kushi's commentary is indicated by the initials* **MK.** *Comments made by former* East West Journal *editor Alex Jack, who sat in on the interview, are indicated by the initials* **AJ.**

## Michio, can you summarize for us the key factors which contribute to the development of cancer?

**MK:** There are many theories today about the cause of cancer, including those of radiation, environmental pollution, heredity, and viruses, as well as certain psychological theories; but practically speaking, with all types of cancer, the basic cause is the day-to-day dietary practices of the individual. These other factors such as radiation and pollution can accelerate the accumulation and spread of cancer, but only if the body is already in a weakened state. The reason that some people would be more susceptible to the effects of radiation, for instance, is that the overall condition of their blood and tissues is not healthy as a result of their long-time dietary habits. Therefore the cancer cannot be changed unless a proper diet is begun.

Originally published in March, 1983 (East West Journal Vol. 13 No. 3)

## Are there certain types of cancer which are more directly affected by diet and others which are more influenced by outside factors?

**MK:** Yes, cancers of the digestive organs, such as stomach or colon cancer, are nearly 100 percent of the time caused by food, but some other cancers like lung cancer can result from a combination of causes. For instance, suppose a person consumes a large amount of animal food along with sugar and chemicals, causing mucus and fat to build up in the body. If this person begins to smoke, it can bring the fat and mucus up into the lungs and cause cancer. A similar example is skin cancer. Sun and radiation definitely can accelerate the creation of skin cancer, but again, the underlying cause is diet.

## Historically, what was the Oriental medical view of cancer? Was there such a term or disease, and how was it treated?

**MK:** Sometimes, around the seashore villages, you would find people who were developing tumors, usually due to eating too much fish and other seafood. If the tumor was near the surface, just under the skin, then sometimes it was operated on, but usually the approach was to semi-fast, to go on a very simple diet of grains, beans, and vegetables with minimal oil and animal food.

Other than that, there was very seldom a development of the disease that we know as cancer. There were a number of symptoms that approximated what we today call cancer, but they were not labelled as a specific disease, and so their symptoms were all treated differently, not just as one illness. This is different from the conventional medical approach today which seems to be looking for one cure for a large number of symptoms that have been grouped together and called cancer.

## How do you define cancer?

**MK:** I would say that it is the ultimate physical self-protection method of the body. The actual process is a localization of the abnormal cells which have been created by excesses of certain kinds of food factors, such as protein and fat.

## In the past, you have said that macrobiotics acts to strengthen the whole body to the point at which the tumor, or cancer, is no longer necessary as a focalizing point for the disease, but now your explanation seems to be more that a macrobiotic diet ac-

**tually dissolves the tumor. Can you explain more specifically how this works?**

**MK:** Yes, when a person starts on a macrobiotic diet, the blood begins to change. As the body is nourished by this new blood, some of the abnormal cells actually change to normal cells, and some abnormal cells die as new ones are created. Let me make an analogy with plants.

The leaves of a plant are like the internal cells in a human body, but they are open, exposed, and more visible. The liquid that passes up through the roots and stem to the leaves is like our blood. This liquid actually becomes the cells of the plant, or organs of the body, so if this liquid is not proper for the plant, then the leaves become misshaped and deformed. However, if the liquid that flows up the stem becomes correct, then either the leaves will change to a more normal form or will die, and new healthy leaves will grow. It is the combination of the liquid and plant together that makes the change.

So, cancer in the body usually localizes in one organ, which is like a leaf on a plant. This is helpful because it is saving millions of other cells. The fact which determines which branch or organ will localize the disease is related to the quality of the excess taken in. For example, excess sugar or dairy foods such as ice cream and milk will localize in the upper parts of the body; animal fats and hard, salty dairy foods like cheese will localize in the lower parts of the body, and a combination will localize in the middle parts of the body.

**What causes cancer to metastasize, that is, spread to other parts of the body?**

**MK:** Cancer will metastasize when excess minerals spill into the blood from the cancerous organ. The excess minerals will either be heavier and denser, such as sodium or calcium from animal and dairy food, or lighter, more diffusive ones such as potassium and sulfur from tropical fruits or vegetables such as potatoes, tomatoes, and avocados.

**What about the psychological aspect of cancer—is there a recognizable cancer personality?**

**MK:** The body and mind are one. If the body gets sick, usually the mental attitude is unhealthy also. The emotional qualities of stubbornness, egocentric thinking, arrogance, fear, hatred, anxiety, or depression are usually accompanied by physical feelings of tiredness, pain, and other minor symptoms of sickness. These two aspects usually develop together toward a cancerous condition.

But in addition to this, we can also recognize two different types of personalities that indicate different kinds of cancerous conditions: one is nourished and cultivated by overconsumption of animal food and very salty foods, and the other is a personality that is developed by overconsumption of sugary foods, soft drinks, and excess fruit. The first type of person is more egocentric, more aggressive, with more outgoing type of character. This type of personality may tend to develop cancer of the prostate, pancreas, or colon. The second type is more reserved, more withdrawn, and isolated from other people. These people do not usually participate in social events and gatherings, and may tend to develop cancer such as leukemia or Hodgkin's disease.

### Would you say, then, that most mental illness is a type of cancer?

**MK:** Yes, usually. Alex, do you have a comment on this?

**AJ:** Yes, there are certain unbalanced psychological states which are fairly accurate indicators of a pre-cancerous condition. For example, if someone demonstrates extreme emotional behavior like acute depression or violent aggressiveness, this person may be developing a cancerous condition as well. Also the breakup of a family, or feelings of always being in conflict with society, warn of a cancerous condition.

### Are you saying that unusual family or environmental situations can increase the risk of cancer?

**AJ:** It is difficult to make a one-to-one link between the specific cause and effect of cancer because these conditions may be leading to other illnesses such as heart disease. All of these conditions—physical, mental, and emotional—that we have been talking about are signs of a degenerating quality of the blood which is the basic means of nourishment for our whole body and mind. So if these early warning signals are not heeded and the person does not change his or her diet and lifestyle, cancer may very well be the end result.

### Are there physical symptoms that indicate a pre-cancerous state?

**MK:** Yes, there are many symptoms that are considered pre-cancerous. No disease arises alone or independent of the whole condition of the body. All sicknesses develop gradually from a less serious stage to a more serious illness. Some examples of conditions that may become more serious if not corrected are constant feelings of fatigue, headaches, frequent urination, or constipation. Others are abnormal vaginal discharge, mucus formation in the body, breast cysts, ovarian cysts, and stone formation in the kidney or gall bladder. At a more progressive stage, skin disorders may occur, such as very dry and flaky skin, freckles, moles, or warts.

**Can all of the visitors you see reverse their cancerous conditions by following the diet you recommend, or are some of them not able to improve their conditions because of family background or situations?**

**MK:** Most of the people I see have been declared medically terminal. Most modern medical approaches have not been able to help them. Also, a majority of them have tried various other alternative methods first, like taking vitamins, or other diets and supplements. Therefore, I would say that only half of my visitors have the physical and mental conditions strong enough to clearly understand the macrobiotic approach, which is to change their dietary and lifestyle patterns.

Of these, half have the desire to change their way of life, but do not develop the proper understanding of the way of cooking to make themselves better. Or they may try the diet with a combination of various other programs which may even make them worse. Of the remaining quarter, some try successfully at first, but may lack family cooperation or the approval of their family doctor which is important to them at this time; so they may eventually return to their original way of life and become ill again.

So this leaves only about 15 to 20 percent among my visitors who are able to get better. If they would come to me at an earlier stage of illness, or had greater family support, the percentage would be much higher.

**Just how important is family support, and what about the feelings of strangeness or isolation a person may feel after starting a macrobiotic diet?**

**MK:** Among some of my visitors, the whole family may attend and they may all want to understand and change their lifestyle along with the person. Such cases usually create very good results. But if a person tries to change alone without his or her family, then that person tends to treat diet as a nutritional therapy for a particular condition, not unlike a standard symptomatic treatment. After they get better, these people easily give up and want to return to a typical standard American diet. However, if that person is patient, and strong enough to take the necessary time to heal, then in two or three years, their family might also try the diet after they see the effect it has.

**It seems that fear often makes a person take the leap of faith to try the macrobiotic approach; but without fear, how can this change be encouraged?**

**MK:** Ah, that is a really big question. A deep study of the macrobiotic understanding of life is needed.

**What advice do you have for people to more easily make a spiritual or mental change in attitude?**

**AJ:** People must change their way of looking at life as well as their way of eating. In our society, we are all subject to consumer attitudes—which means that we expect instant results. If we don't see an immediate change, we usually discard that practice and go on to something else. So if someone tries macrobiotics with the attitude that it is like an instant pill or drug, and they don't get the instant fulfillment they expect, then they may go on to another way of life. These mental and spiritual outlooks need to be changed—we need to be willing to take inspiration from the natural world in which growth and change is slow and organic like the food we eat. We have to allow this in the healing process and realize that this change is going to be for the rest of our lives, not just a one-year situation. Food is the basis for this healing, which then affects our emotions, our thoughts, and our spiritual development.


**MK:** I would like to add that this approach is not symptomatic like taking pills or having surgery. This approach is the self-curing method. In that sense, the person with cancer has to make a psychologically and spiritually deep self-reflection of what he or she has done. That person must admit that the food that has been consumed and the previous lifestyle are what led to his or her present condition. The decision must then be made to change the way of life along with diet. Therefore this approach is comprehensive. Psychological, spiritual, and emotional factors must all be taken together.

**It seems to be the common medical assumption that when one has a serious illness such as cancer, it is not time to go on a special diet and risk malnutrition. Can you comment on that?**

**MK:** Most doctors think from the view of nutritional elements, instead of how humans can re-adapt themselves to be in harmony with nature. Our approach is to decide what food is best to develop good humanity.

**But is it possible to become malnourished on the diet?**

**MK:** No, not if it is being practiced with the proper understanding—a macrobiotic diet contains all necessary nutrients. Also, the macrobiotic diet is not a limited, static approach. It should always be changing with the person's needs and condition; so if malnutrition begins, then a modification is necessary. This is the macrobiotic way.

**Is it possible for a sick person to cook for him- or herself and still get better?**

**MK:** Yes, however, in the event that one cannot think for oneself, it is better first to be fed by someone, or guided by someone. The more one eats this way, the more one's thinking and understanding will gradually improve.

**Once people are declared medically relieved of cancer, are they totally cured as whole individuals, or is there more to it?**

**MK:** As I mentioned before, there must be a psychological change as well. The first stage is symptom relief. Medically, this may be called a cure, however, this is actually just the beginning. Mental processes and social behavior may not necessarily be corrected. The person may begin again to practice the wrong way of life and eating and thereby again attract cancer or another degenerative disease.

I can make three suggestions to help change the mental attitude more quickly: first we must relax and cease to struggle with ourselves. A reliance on our natural healing processes must be felt. We must realize that we need not to worry, but rather feel a submission, a giving of ourselves to the Universe, and trust that everything will be taken care of. Secondly, we can look around us and notice how everything in our surroundings is supported and nourished by every other part of nature. In this way, we can become grateful and learn how to appreciate everything in our environment. Thirdly, if we try to return to others what we owe, and do everything for others that we can, then this is the experience of love.

**AJ:** Actually, if a person who develops cancer still has a relatively clear mental condition as the result of a basically strong constitution, then he may come to look at his illness as the most important experience in his life. He may appreciate the cancer for what it has taught him about the nature of his life and the order of nature in the larger perspective. He may begin to recognize that all positive and negative experiences balance and complement each other. In this way, the cancer becomes his friend, a teacher that can produce a change in consciousness in the spiritual dimension which we discussed earlier.

### What about other therapies such as herbs, Laetrile, visualization, or the raw foods diet? Are some of these compatible with macrobiotics?

**MK:** Alex, can you comment on this?

**AJ:** These alternative therapies have mixed results. In some cases they seem to relieve symptoms, and in other cases there are no visible effects. Sometimes there can be very negative effects. The reason is that these treatments do not take into account that cancer is caused by a number of different factors. It does not have one single origin, but comes from an extreme imbalance in one of two general directions, the more contracted condition resulting from the overconsumption of animal products and foods that are too salty, or the more expanded condition coming from refined foods and sugars. So, therefore, trying to heal cancer with just one specific factor, whether it is wheatgrass, raw foods, or pancreatic enzymes, may have some positive effect on one condition, but can have a disastrous effect if taken by someone with the opposite condition. For instance, with Laetrile, which is derived from a fruit—the pit of an apricot—people with the first type of cancer from an excess of hard, salty animal foods will tend to respond because the treatment creates a balance with their condition. However, if people with leukemia or Hodgkin's disease tried this treatment, it would tend to accelerate their tumorous development. This is one of the reasons that the medical profession tends to dismiss these therapies—there are very mixed results.

### Are there any other recommendations within the macrobiotic approach besides diet that you offer to the person with cancer?

**MK:** Yes, I always advise my visitors to scrub their bodies with a moist towel every day to accelerate blood and energy circulation, as well as physical and mental metabolism. Also, I advise practically everyone to do some exercise, again to revitalize their whole metabolism. I also suggest that they make order in their immediate surroundings, avoiding synthetic materials, especially in clothes directly next to the skin, and to limit or avoid watching television or working under white fluorescent lights. I also recommend avoiding the use of electricity, especially for cooking. Microwave cooking should never be used. Next, I often urge visitors to establish good relations with their parents and families, and in some cases I recommend meditation, or deep-breathing exercise, for a total lifestyle approach.

### Is collaboration with a medical doctor necessary, or harmful, or doesn't it make any difference?

**MK:** I think, generally, we recommend that keeping the hospital or doctor informed of the dietary approach and trying to work in harmony with them would be beneficial, especially in terms of keeping medical records and reports.

### What about combining the treatments recommended by the doctor with the macrobiotic approach?

**MK:** When I have a conference with medical doctors, I always advise that the patient should change his diet immediately. Then, if the medical view is that the modern approach is necessary, they may continue to use it for a while, but all doctors and patients know that although these medical approaches can sometimes work to relieve symptoms, in most cases they will at the same time bring the patient to a very weak condition. Therefore medical treatment should be very well supervised, and not over-used. However, if the dietary approach is working by itself, then it is better to refrain from medical treatment.

### Can this approach be learned from a book, or do people have to go to a teacher?

**MK:** The macrobiotic approach is primarily a person's intuitive, common-sense approach. However, at the present time, modern people seem to have lost that common sense, so, until they rediscover and reactivate it, they need to be guided by experienced persons. At the same time, they should study, read books, or attend classes and seminars. However, the eventual goal of macrobiotics is to achieve an understanding of how to maintain one's own health.

## Is the macrobiotic approach to cancer expensive?

**MK:** No, the macrobiotic approach is very economical. Each individual food item may seem somewhat higher in price than similar items because of the more natural processes by which it is made and its organic quality; however, because of reduction of animal food and sugar consumption, daily food costs will become one-third or less. This is not even to mention what can be saved on medical expenses. Recently, in meetings with my visitors, I was amazed to learn that among eight of them, there had been around eighty operations. The total that they had spent as a group came to nearly half a million dollars. This included hospital expenses, drugs, and surgery in a span of about eight to ten years. Therefore, on the whole, I should certainly say that the dietary approach I recommend is much more economical for the individual, for society, for the country, and for the whole world.

## Why are there not more statistics on cases of cancer relief due to macrobiotics?

**MK:** This is actually the beginning of a new phase for the East West Foundation [the organization in Boston which distributes information about cancer and diet]. We have never performed any medical procedures such as blood tests, so there have been no records.

For the past fifteen years, we have been working without the thought of making this statistical information available, but now we realize that we must change as there is a growing demand for this type of information. I have always felt that this is a revolutionary way of healing sickness, so we have been more concerned with helping people than keeping records.

## What do you think it will take for macrobiotics to become more widely accepted, instead of just another alternative approach?

**MK:** We need to de-mystify the words used in macrobiotics and use common Western terminology. In this way, we can show that this is not really a strange approach, but just common-sense principles that we all use anyway, knowingly or unknowingly.

Along with this, there should be a study of the larger view of life and the universal principles of relativity. If we can understand this and learn to express it consciously in our approach to diet and health, then it can begin to make a significant difference in the total approach to sickness and disease. We should also use this understanding to explain other conditions as well, such as our economic, social, and ideologic attitudes. Then we can begin to see that this approach is not an "alternative," but includes everything.

Macrobiotics will eventually be the guideline for future generations. It can act as a compass to help us solve many and various difficulties. It does not just cure sickness but helps to realize the absolute maximum health, happiness, and spiritual freedom for an individual. This in turn will create one happy peaceful world—a planet on which we can play from morning to night.

Cancer is just a speck, one small finger of macrobiotics. We will now graduate from this level to other levels of play. We already know it is helpful and effective for the relief of cancer if done properly, so now we can turn to the larger issues of peace, crime, mental illness, and world hunger.

### What advice can you offer Western medical doctors in their research on disease?

**MK:** Mainly, I would recommend to them to study the "macro" view of health and sickness, instead of always the "micro" world under a microscope. They should try to find out the cause of disease on the level of cells and molecules, and see how that relates to the larger view.

I hope that medicine and nutrition can develop along with an understanding also of astronomy, economics, environmental issues, agriculture, and an awareness of how present lifestyles affect our nutritional values.

### What books would you recommend that someone read to gain an understanding of this?

**MK:** Unfortunately, no colleges teach this type of information yet, but any of the classical books dealing with humanity's relationship to God and the Universe would be good to read. The words used in macrobiotics have roots in traditional Western texts as well as Eastern. The Greeks talked about the art of healthful eating and being in tune with the harmony of nature. Georges Ohsawa did not invent the word macrobiotics. It was also used by the Greeks. These are traditional human words. Some good books to study would be Hippocrates, the fragments of Heracles, and other pre-Socratic texts, along with more modern works by Samuel Butler, Edward Carpenter, Ralph Waldo Emerson, Alexis Carrel, and F.S.C. Northrup.

**Do you have any other final words to say about the use of macrobiotics in relieving cancer?**

**MK:** Yes, I would like to say that I appreciate modern medicine's efforts to deal with cancer and degenerative disease and I will be continually grateful if we can work together. I appreciate very much the U.S. Government's Dietary Goals that were published in 1977, as well as other work of various other public institutions, such as the Heart Association and the U.S. Department of Agriculture; also the recent National Academy of Science's reports recommending a correction of dietary patterns by increasing the consumption of grains, vegetables, and beans, and decreasing the intake of animal and dairy foods. I also appreciate the great number of macrobiotic people throughout the world who have begun to work for natural agriculture, food processing, and establishing natural foods industries. Because of these joint efforts, I have an optimistic opinion regarding the future of health in the world.

# II
# POLITICS

# 6

# United States Food Policy

*One September 21, 1977, Michio Kushi and representatives of the macrobiotic com-munity met in Washington with members of the executive branch involved in President Jimmy Carter's reorganization of food policy. The government officials were presented with the macrobiotic viewpoint on food issues, ranging from agriculture to nutrition and health. The meeting, which lasted approximately two hours, began with a forty-five minute presentation of statements by macrobiotic leaders including the following recommendations by Michio Kushi.*

## INTRODUCTION

In the United States as well as in other modern nations over the past few decades, people have been experiencing the effects of the biological and sociological degeneration of humanity. The tendency toward this degeneration includes the following aspects:

1.  increase of chronic physical degenerative illness among people in all walks of life (e.g., arthritis, heart disease, cancer, etc.);
2.  increase of psychological illness among people in all walks of life;
3.  increase of uncontrollable behavior, especially among children and the younger generation;
4.  increase in the abuse of hallucinogenic drugs and the so-called "mood-altering" prescription drugs (e.g., tranquilizers, stimulants, depressants, etc.)
5.  decline in the working efficiency of people at all levels of employment and increasing loss of work-time due to illness;

Originally published in November, 1977 (East West Journal Vol. 7 No. 11)

6. decline in young people's spirit of respect for traditional values and the older generation, along with a decline in parents' direct love for children and the younger generation, appearing in its extreme form as mounting cases of physical abuse;

7. general decomposition of harmonious family unity;

8. increase in the crime rate including violent crimes, especially among younger people.

If this widespread degenerative tendency continues to accelerate at its present rate for another two decades, American society will face serious impairment of its economic, political, social, religious, educational, and cultural vitality.

Having examined this physical, mental, and social trend for over twenty years, we have come to the conclusion that the major cause of this general phenomenon lies in what the majority of individuals and families consume daily through their present dietary practice.

Accordingly, we have devoted ourselves for the past twenty years to educational activities in order to promote a better understanding of healthy food, including its production, processing, preparation, and consumption. Our educational activities, involving lectures, seminars, publications, and personal contact, have contributed to promoting a trend toward the natural food movement in the United States as well as several countries in South America and Europe.

As a whole, those people who have followed our dietary recommendations have recovered through their own efforts a more vital and sounder way of life, regaining their physical, mental, and spiritual health, as well as developing more efficient study and work habits. For documentation, please consult the *Case History Reports*, available from the East West Foundation (17 Station Street, Brookline, MA 02147), which include reports on recovery from the following problems:

1. cancer, arthritis, epilepsy, heart disease, skin diseases, chronic digestive troubles, general fatigue, and other physical problems;

2. mental fatigue, depression, anxiety, fear, and other psychological disorders;

3. misunderstanding and quarreling within families, including problems of the so-called generation gap;

4. disrespect for the traditional values and spirit of hardworking ancestors;

5.   chaotic and disorderly lifestyles;
6.   abuse of hallucinogenic drugs.

## RECOMMENDATIONS

As a practical way to reverse the present degenerative trend in national health, we would recommend the following general policies:

1.   In order to preserve the natural health-building quality of food, there should be no—or at least far fewer—chemicals used in the production and processing of food. The current over-refinement and other extremely artificial treatment of foods should be gradually reduced as much as possible.
2.   Agriculture should gradually shift from the current style of artificial mass production to a more natural style of production, in order to restore natural quality.
3.   Food preparation should become more family-style, re-emphasizing the kitchen in every home as the site of most cooking rather than mass preparation—in particular, in the current highly commercial "pre-packaged" and "fast food" style.
4.   Food for daily consumption should consist of two basic categories: principal food and supplementary food, along the following lines:

     The principal staple to be unrefined, whole cereal grains and their products. They should constitute approximately 50 percent or more of the daily intake. Examples of such foods are: whole wheat, brown rice, oats, barley, rye, millet, corn, and buckwheat, in all their forms (such as bread, pasta, porridge, pancakes, crackers, biscuits, etc.).

     The supplementary food to include several categories which should vary according to regional and seasonal environmental conditions as well as personal needs. Examples of such foods are vegetables, beans, seaweeds, fruits, seeds and nuts, moderate quantities of fish and other seafood, poultry and eggs (on occasion).

     In general, artificial beverages and highly aromatic, stimulant foods and drinks are not recommended for daily consumption. The current heavy reliance on meat, mass-produced, nonfertilized eggs, and highly refined or industrially treated food products and drinks is also to be discouraged. The current heavy consumption of dairy food is to be reduced. Such foods should be recommended only if they have been processed in a way that keeps the natural quality through traditional methods. Reliance on sugar and similar mono-and disaccharide sweeteners should be replaced by shifting to polysaccharide sweets, mainly processed from grains and vegetables.

5.  In addition to food composition, proper selection of good quality food and proper cooking of these foods is also important. We recommend sea salt for cooking instead of highly refined, mined salt, and cold-pressed, pure quality vegetable oil instead of chemically and high-temperature-processed oil. For seasoning and to aid digestion of grains, we recommend traditional foods such as naturally fermented soybean products (e.g., soy sauce, miso, tempeh, etc.) and pickled vegetables.

6.  We recommend a return to the traditional custom of families cooking and eating together at least once a day, in order to assure each family's health and to strengthen mutual understanding among family members as well as family friends.

The cost of food for the diet recommended here is approximately one-third the cost of present dietary patterns, yet through this traditional way of eating all daily nutritional requirements are met as well as and, in fact, much more easily than with the present American diet. This financial saving alone could be of great help in recovering the sound economic condition of individual families and society as a whole.

## NATIONAL BENEFITS

If the United States reorients its food goals in a direction similar to that proposed here, many major aspects of various social problems would eventually be resolved considerably. The social benefits resulting from such a policy would include the following areas:

1.  The general health of the American public will become much sounder. This improvement could save enormous amounts of money on every level from family, community, city, and state to federal. Expenditures saved on health care could be used for more productive and creative uses.

2. Schools and other educational facilities can function much more smoothly as a result of students and teachers recovering their native intellectual and emotional balance.

3. The rate of crimes, including violent acts, will decrease substantially, resulting in a much safer, less fear-ridden, and more peaceful society, as well as a very substantial saving of money currently spent on police and legal procedures.

4. Divorce and the breakup of families, as well as general conflicts in human relations, will decrease significantly. Naturally caring relationships will eventually be restored throughout society, leading to happier personal and community life as a whole. This easing of current tensions between individuals and between social groups will reduce the present need for governmental regulatory control of the people.

5. All private enterprises, companies, institutions, and public organizations will benefit from the increased efficiency that comes from the recovery of sound physical and mental health in people. This change will ensure the future of the country in the direction of greater prosperity.

6. The population that the country is able to support comfortably will be substantially increased as direct consumption of grains replaces the current wasteful pattern of consuming these products indirectly in the form of animal food; currently overgrazed land will also become arable again.

## TRANSITION PROGRAMS

There are, of course, enormous problems which must be solved in order to achieve the goal of the above recommendations. It cannot be expected that the above recommendations could be put into practice in a short period of time. We estimate that it will take approximately twenty years before the majority of the United States could shift in this general direction. In the meantime, all our efforts, public and personal, should be directed to the following concerns:

1. The clear and unified reorientation of government agencies toward a new policy on food and agriculture should be designed within a reasonably short period of time.

2. A program of education for food producers—including farmers, processors and manufacturers—should be designed with the goal of producing better, more natural food, with the assistance, where possible, of federal, state, and local agencies. These educational programs should involve conventions, conferences, seminars, publications, and the media.

3. The staffs of schools, hospitals, hotels, restaurants, airlines, and other public eating places should be educated in the use of better-quality food and better application of cooking methods, avoiding as much as possible synthetic, chemicalized, and overly-refined foods and beverages. Such education can also be promoted through conferences, conventions, lectures, discussions, and publication of booklets.

4. Families, as well as individuals, should be educated about good food. Such education could be spread through lectures, conferences, and discussions with women's associations, community organizations, and social clubs, as well as adult education. Magazines, newspapers, television, and other media should also be asked to participate.

5. In this connection, establishing a public educational team for community health resembling the "Peace Corps" might be considered. The education and training of such community workers may take six months to one year prior to actually beginning their educational services in society. Education for the members of a community health service should include:

   a. general theories of nutrition, modern and traditional, and the relationship of diet to major physical and mental disorders;

   b. difference in the techniques and results of organic, non-chemicalized agriculture compared to artificial, energy-intensive agricultural (including field visits):

   c. practical study of food selection and cooking until the participants are qualified to advise individuals and families (some members may become capable of offering advice on the way of cooking in public eating places such as restaurants and hotels, as well as institutional eating places);

   d. study of practical methods of simple food processing (such as baking, pickling, etc.) for home use;

   e. understanding of governmental regulations related to foods and beverages;

   f. learning practical family counseling.

6.  Medical practitioners also should be encouraged to recommend proper food to patients as a standard part of therapy. Education of medical professionals is recommended on the relationship between food and disease. Such information can be included not only in the educational programs of fully accredited medical schools, as well as lectures, seminars, discussions, and conferences for medical professionals and paraprofessionals.

## CONCLUSIONS

A shift from the present dietary trends in the United States toward a healthier and sounder direction will result in improved economic welfare for the country. A sizeable portion of the agricultural products of the nation, including grains, beans, and seaweeds, can be exported to other countries which presently suffer from general malnutrition. This policy will also lower the cost of living and public expenditures; it will substantially lower food costs, medical expenses, Social Security and Welfare expenses; and it will improve people's working efficiency. It can be foreseen that our country will develop in this way towards a healthy, peaceful, intellectual, happier, and more prosperous future. This shift, however, should be neither radical nor unreasonably fast. It should proceed in gradual steps within every community and industry, as producers, suppliers, and consumers are able to adapt. Accordingly, educational services for the above-described areas should be conducted very actively.

# 7

## Michio Kushi's New Deal The Coming World Government

### How did you first become interested in world government?

The times in which I grew up were unusually strained, not only in Japan but throughout the world. International relations were very tense, due to economic and military competition all over the globe. The major powers were building huge armies, and most economies were geared to that purpose. At the same time, general education for everyone was slanted according to that orientation of militarism. Finally war broke out, worldwide. It was that experience that marked me so deeply.

In the war so many people died, including, of course, many of my friends. I myself was drafted and went through many war experiences. In personal terms, such tense, extreme situations can actually be very beneficial on the physical and spiritual level in that they develop strength, judgment, and so forth. Sufferings, poverty—both serve that purpose. But on the social level of the whole world, it was a time of nightmare. That was the cause of my interest in world peace.

### How did you begin working for that?

At first, at the end of World War II, I thought of working on the existing world political structures. I felt that if some kind of world government could enforce law on the international level, resolving relationships between countries and the major power blocs, then that would relieve world tension. Those relationships include freedom of communication, questions of a just food distribution, free immigration, control of atomic energy and other energy sources, etc. It seemed to many people at that

Originally published in January, 1976 (East West Journal Vol. 6 No. 1)

time that such a world government could be achieved by amending the charter of the United Nations.

Another approach was to bypass the United Nations entirely—since it is an organization based on the concept of national sovereignty—and to set up independently a world congress as the basis of a planetary government that would represent the people of the whole world. The representatives would be nongovernmental people—students and so forth. That civil body would then appeal to the governments of each nation and would thus serve as a place where the people of the world, regardless of nationality, could begin to create a world government.

Although opinion varied on the best form for world government to take, many people at that time were very interested in the issue. Gandhi, Einstein, Thomas Mann, Upton Sinclair, Norman Cousins, and many other leaders wanted to achieve the goal of world government, but on a practical level it seemed almost impossible to proceed.

I went to talk with many of the leaders in this movement such as Thomas Mann, Albert Einstein, and others. At that time I was a graduate student in international law at Columbia University. I also studied this problem at Harvard and with the Quakers. Finally I began to realize that a change in structure, which was what everyone was seeking, would not be sufficient. It wasn't really the whole solution but only a symptomatic remedy, and therefore it couldn't actually work in the long run. It's true, of course, that if we organized a powerful world government, we might be able to halt major international war, but people's suffering and civil strife arising from all sorts of unhappiness, sickness, and so forth would still exist; our underlying problem would not be solved.

What is basically necessary, then, in order to create one happy, peaceful world? The basic question is how all people can develop freedom, health, and happiness on the individual level. How can they really evolve, psychologically and physiologically? That question is the subject matter of macrobiotics, the study of the Unifying Principle. As you know, that Unifying Principle deals with yin and yang, or balance, as the basic order of the universe on all levels—spiritual, social, individual, biochemical, and so on.

**You say that macrobiotics is the way to solve the question of how all people can live together in peace. But Jesus also thought that his way would work. Buddha thought his method was the answer. In fact, every guru says that about his own**

**system. Even people who take EST think that's the answer. All these movements and religions throughout history have said they had the answer, and they have all failed. Why do you think your answer is different? What is the reason for your saying that macrobiotics will finally bring world peace?**

Macrobiotics means living in harmony with the order of the universe. Whoever ignores that holistic view of constant change and is exlusive or rigid, taking macrobiotics as a particular method or a set belief system which is the only way as opposed to various other systems, may call himself macrobiotic, but that is not really macrobiotics. Macrobiotics is always striving for the large view and must never be fragmentary or partial. The various approaches of different teachings and religions are included in a truly macrobiotic view; they are not excluded, as if macrobiotics were one particular way, like a special religion or movement. Macrobiotics studies these different approaches, trying to see the cause of each, its dynamic mechanism, what level it appeals to, what kind of future it has, its strengths and limitations. It strives to see every phenomenon in terms of front and back, yin and yang, always investigating balance, wholeness. So it does not deny or reject any approach.

**Most people think of macrobiotics as a diet, yet what you describe is much more than that. How would you define macrobiotics?**

Eating the proper food ecologically is, of course, important. Without health there can be no peace, so the first step is to restore our harmony and oneness with our total surroundings. But the next step is to study the dynamic mechanism of all phenomena, not only diet, but psychology, education, politics, economics, etc. In order to truly understand a problem, we must see the "how" of it. Through that understanding, we can cope with any situation and establish harmony in our lives. That is macrobiotics.

**Many people who read the *East West Journal* are interested in meditation and also in developing alternative lifestyles including natural food. Many of them seem to feel that concentrating on building an alternative to the present materialistic society is enough to change the world into a more harmonious**

**system than we see around us presently. How do you see the evolution of that process?**

We can perhaps use Hegel's dialectic of thesis, antithesis and synthesis. Many present ideals of alternative ways are reactions to the conventional way. The two exist as thesis and antithesis, balancing each other; the existing of the one depends on the existence of the other. That is a temporary situation rather than a comprehensive synthesis.

The embracing answer is not in reaction but in firmly establishing our total harmony with nature and the universe. As that springs from our physiological and psychological health, we begin at the same time to structure a harmonious society. That harmonious society may have some alternative elements, some conventional elements, perhaps some elements from the prehistoric world, and some entirely new, visionary elements. It would not be just alternatives, as a reaction.

**What would world government be in such a society?**

A harmonious world government would differ from present government, especially in two essentials. First, it should be essentially a service organization, rather than a governing organization; second, the representatives in such an organization should include two types of people, yin and yang. Present governments include only yang people, active types of people interested in power rather than meditation or spiritual approaches.

**How could yin people be included in government?**

By the recommendation of the people. Yin people—like, for example, sages in the older societies—aren't the kind of people who speak up for themselves, saying "I want to run for president." So the people must recommend them. Also, it would help for the inclusion of such yin people if the process of choosing representatives included not only speeches but also more written material, since yin people are often better writers and yang people better speakers. There should also be more representation of women's voice.

**What do you see developing in this direction during the next twenty-five years?**

Over the next twenty-five years, existing institutions will generally go into an increasingly rapid decline. At the same time, the alternative movment will spread, but will tend to take many different forms, rapidly shifting from one plan to another. Meanwhile, macrobiotics will spread, establishing a large popular base of healthy people who are ready to cooperate and share in creating a harmonious world government. In my opinion, true world government cannot be imposed as a structure from the top, but must arise from the natural readiness of everyone. That will take many, many years of natural growth.

## How many?

About two thousand.

## Why?

First, because of conditions developing on the earth as a planet, as I discussed in my articles on the Ancient and Future Worlds *(see chapters 13 and 14—ed.)* with regard to the precession of the equinox and its effect on human life. Secondly, I am counting the rate of growth of macrobiotics (allowing for dropouts of course) figuring children, children's children, and so forth.

## In the future society you describe, would there be a world currency, and would it be based on gold?

Not gold, people's trust. The natural resources of the whole earth would back up the value of that currency. But that value depends on people's working ability—thus, in that sense, people's trust. When people's health and psychological confidence decline, the value of currency depreciates.

## What about energy in the future? Presently, energy resources are managed by centralized organizations, and we rely on forms of energy whose development requires enormous capital, which is available only to huge organizations.

Our energy should not come from deposited sources, fossil fuels. That is living off our capital in the earth instead of the interest produced by natural growth. We should use the energy that constantly comes down to the earth from the universe, and also the energy that is constantly generated from the earth out toward the universe—that is, centrifugal force. We should shift to these more basic energies, which exist on the electromagnetic level rather than the visible, material level. Those universal kinds of energy are totally undeveloped, yet they are tremendous, causing the earth's rotation, the evolution of the solar system, and the motion of the stars.

Also, basic energies should be the kind of energy that can't be monopolized by one economic group or country. Their nature is such that they belong to everyone living on the earth; the world's people own them.

**So you wouldn't need huge factories or industrial complexes to develop it?**

That's right. And not only should energy be possessed by all the people in common; all the basics such as land and essential food should really be free. It will take time, however, to realize that the present way of paying for things to an owner is an illusion. Of course, extras—like a car, if you want to have one—can be owned as private property. However, the world government, as a service organization, should assure that the basics belong to everyone.

**That will only come, however, when people, by and large, are no longer interested in owning things—such as energy, food, land—that are now considered the key to power.**

Right. So people must still go through another twenty or thirty years of fighting over those things until they wake up to the contradictions of that system.

**Recently you've started to travel, especially to Europe, giving lecture tours there, after having lived and taught in America for twenty-five years. Is there any specific reason or timetable behind that sequence?**

Yes. I spent my first ten years in this country as my training: experiencing American customs, doing all kinds of different work, being exposed to many ideas, etc. For the next fifteen years, I taught macrobiotics. Now I can see that America's fundamental physiological revolution is firmly underway. There's no longer any stopping it. The trend cannot reverse itself back toward chemicalized, refined foods. The movement toward natural, organic foods has gathered momentum. Food can only become sounder and better and better now.

So the first step, regaining our health, is now practically accomplished; it's only a matter of time. The second step, education for understanding, however, involves not only America but also Europe, since America and Europe form one ideological cultural unit, "modern Western civilization." To establish that second level—the ideological, psychological transformation following the physiological revolution—Europe must change as well. That's why I'm teaching in Europe.

Tracing the problems to their origin, the sequence goes this way: in order to change the Far East, where I grew up, America must be transformed. In order for America to be transformed, ideologically, Europe must also change. In order for Europe to change, the Slavic bloc and Asia must change. So the origin is always traceable toward the East, geographically. However, the principal area now is the Western bloc of America and Europe, because the whole world—Asia, Africa, South America—is now imitating the ways of modern Western civilization.

**I've heard the word macrobiotics used to describe three different groups of people. First, it refers to people who have switched from the modern diet of meat, dairy food, sugar, and refined foods to whole grains and cooked vegetables as the staple of their diet and who have begun to study phenomena in terms of yin and yang; however, in relating to the rest of the world, this first group of people has a tendency to act self-righteous and exclusive, which is contrary to the all-embracive philosophy that you said is the essence of macrobiotics. Second, many traditional cultures throughout the world—for example, the Hunzas or the Vilcabambas, whose diet is in harmony with their natural environment and who live long, happy lives full of respect for the perennial values such as humility, joyfulness, responsibility, etc.—are also said to be macrobiotic. The third group of people who have been called macrobiotic includes certain great individuals, such as Benjamin Franklin and Thomas Jefferson in America, who led very active lives mentally and physically while following a moderate vegetarian or semi-vegetarian diet and also exemplified the macrobiotic values of endless curiosity that you mentioned earlier. Now, where are the real macrobiotics? I don't see how it can be the first group, since they generally behave just like any other believers in a religion or ideological institution, whereas you said that macrobiotics is not a particular movement but is essentially embracive.**

As I said, macrobiotics is not a special group or religion. Macrobiotics does not dictate to individuals any doctrines or set pattern of behavior that they are supposed to follow as a limitation on their abilities or their own direction. Rather, macrobiotics is the way to develop your own capacities fully and realize your own dream endlessly, through a peaceful, universal type of mentality. It offers people the tools with which to find their direction and follow it. Macrobiotics provides a universal compass, yin and yang, like north and south. A compass tells you which way is north, wherever you are, but what direction you want to take is up to your free judgment. You can become an angel or a devil, as you wish. Harmony has not been established in the world by government, because government has been designed with the goal that only the angels should exist. Real harmony means angels and devils coexisting. Front and back must always be free to coexist.

Your third group, great individuals, can be called macrobiotic in one sense, but the problem is that their character was the result of their excellent constitution and upbringing. So they were created, rather than self-created. They were very fortunate in the parents and early environment they happened to have. They didn't know why they had those wonderful qualities, why they possessed the strong will which enabled them to develop themselves. Since they didn't understand that question, they were not totally in possession of their freedom. Macrobiotics gives people the ability to exercise their full freedom to become whatever they want, great or weak, happy or unhappy, according to their own free will.

The second category you mentioned, traditional culture, suffers from the same kind of difficulty as the third group, great individuals. Although they do live in harmony with nature and the universe, they are not aware of the value of that, in the sense of knowing the why and how behind their harmonious lifestyle. They eventually must re-evaluate their culture in those terms. If they have not done that, then when a new culture, such as modern industrial civilization, comes along with its glamour, they easily succumb. That has been the story with the whole non-Western world, which is now in turmoil.

The first group of people you mentioned, students of macrobiotics, are in a preliminary stage, getting ready to become truly macrobiotic in this fully developed sense of being able to exercise freedom. They are still at the stage of cultivating their health and judgment toward freedom, which they will actually be able to start realizing in its true all-embracing, nonexclusive sense when their health and judgment are more soundly established.

## How exactly can macrobiotics lead to world government? Would you be more specific?

True world government is not an extension of government as we know it. This kind of service-oriented, educational government has never been tried in recorded history. By "educational" I mean not only exchanging information freely but also emphasizing full discussion of the main principles: What is life? What is its purpose? What is happiness? Here also, people must be allowed to follow their own free judgment, not forced to be angels.

Real government is nothing but the order of the universe itself. Present institutional government is actually created to disturb, or interfere with, that natural, marvelous order. We must study that repressive mechanism and learn how government could function instead to liberate people's potential to work freely, manifesting the order of the universe.

Macrobiotics creates an evolutionary change in humanity, a truly free, self-created species of beings able to choose their lives completely on their own. Macrobiotics is the way of freedom. No system can establish that. The only purpose of government is giving freedom to everyone, which has nothing to do with what government now is. It's completely new, waiting to be invented. True world government is a reflection of the glory and everlasting order of the universe. In that sense, the purpose of world government is ultimately to demolish all government as it exists. You may call such true world government "nongovernment"; it will appear only after generations of change toward establishing our own health and judgment.

# 8

## Armageddon

**There's a growing general feeling that somehow the world is coming to an end. What do you think of that?**

Taking a large view, we are influenced by the cosmological order which can be described as the celestial influence upon us. At the present time, we are entering into some kind of definite change on that level. In terms of human history since the birth of *Homo sapiens*, one major era is now ending and a new epoch is beginning.

That change is represented in human society by two types of civilization: a more spiritually oriented and a more materially oriented civilization. Those two tendencies have alternated for the past 300,000 to 400,000 years. For the past five or six thousand years the more materialistic orientation has predominated on the earth. Before that, the more spiritual orientation was in the ascendancy.

During the remainder of this century and the early part of the next century, the shift from material leadership to spiritual leadership will take place. In fact from the late nineteenth century, we can see the spiritual principle beginning to emerge again at the forefront of human thought—for example, the shift in modern physics from a materialistic view to an understanding of particles as nothing but energy—and in general leadership that emphasizes material superiority is losing its credibility and rapidly decaying. That decay will continue in various social phenomena, such as growing chaos in the economic system and increasing upsets in international relations through basic political and economic conflicts. National economics around the world have already begun to encounter very serious difficulties. Furthermore, the familiar

Originally published in January, 1977 (East West Journal Vol. 7 No. 1)

cultural and religious teachings expressed through institutions such as the churches and schools are losing their authority or influence over people. The whole of modern society, which has been oriented in the direction of economics and materialism, will start to disintegrate. Even science has been losing its authority. Unless it is synthesized with a more spiritual, intuitive understanding, it, too, will die out.

Finally, at this time, as a result of the decrease in simple holistic understanding that has marred the last few thousand years, many individuals have become sick and will pass away through degenerative diseases such as mental illness, cancer, heart disease, drug abuse, and so on.

### What major social and political trend do you see developing in terms of these changes?

At the present time, the world is gradually differentiating into two camps: the first includes those who continue on the materially oriented trends of the past few thousand years; the second group is reflecting seriously upon that record and starting to change their way of life and their way of thinking toward a more spiritually oriented civilization. At the base of those two groups, there is developing a subtle but very deep biological difference.

Physiology ultimately expresses what is taken into the organism in the form of food to become the body. Materially oriented civilization promotes, through modern nutritional theories, the consumption of commercialized, chemicalized, mass-produced food. People oriented toward a more spiritual direction, however, tend to select and prefer food that grows more naturally; they create their physiological balance through their own native, common-sense judgment and tend to improve their health. The first group is slowly dying out from chronic, degenerative diseases, as we see now every day. The second group though prone to make some initial mistakes will gradually establish their biological strength and build a new civilization.

For that second group, concepts such as the modern nation state and other artificial assumptions of materialistic society will have no appeal. Rather, the second group will understand that we are all descended from the infinite universe and are born in a natural way as the manifestation of the order of the universe, or you may say in traditional religion terminology, we are the children of God, like brothers and sisters.

## Do you see any reference to this process in Biblical prophecies?

These are many interpretations of the Book of Revelations. The idea behind that work is not only a Christian view; it has existed from more ancient times. The Orient had similar ideas. The description in the Book of Revelations of coming events is actually based upon the celestial motions which I mentioned, not mystical events. The symbols refer to the changing constellations through which the pole star moves during the cycle of the precession of the equinoxes. The Book of Revelations is a description of human destiny as it is influenced by the cycle of northern celestial motion, the 25,800-year cycle of the precession of the equinoxes (*for a fuller explanation, see chapters 13 and 14—ed.*). In that cycle—depending on how the earth's axis is aligned relative to the plane of our galaxy—we alternate between a very prosperous, spiritually oriented time and a troubled, materially oriented time. At the present stage, with the shift to Polaris in Ursa Minor as the new north star, materially oriented society is being superseded by the spiritually oriented society. That transition process is accompanied, of course, by much turmoil. But this turmoil is not caused by mystical factors; it is caused rather by the too narrow view of materialistic thinking which lacks understanding of the larger order of the universe—in this case, the greater celestial cycles. Therefore, if we understand those laws of the universe (which are nothing but the laws of nature) and if we start to live according to them, this turmoil can actually be avoided very smoothly.

As I said, since the nineteenth century there has been growing turmoil—economic, scientific, medical, religious—as many established institutions and familiar beliefs about reality have fallen into question. People rigidly dependent on those belief systems get confused and depressed. For people who are working to live in adaptable harmony with the order of nature, the order of the universe, these changes do not represent turmoil at all. Rather, they are perceived as a kind of necessary purification or adjustment to enable our world to return to a harmonious state.

When most people—especially very fundamentalist Christians—interpret the Book of Revelations, they tend to mystify it by picturing dead souls arising and salvation coming miraculously down from heaven and so forth. These images from the Bible, however, are actually only poetic kinds of descriptions as in mythological accounts; they are for dramatic effect and are not to be taken literally.

**Almost 95 percent of the earthquakes, tidal waves, and similar natural catastrophes over the past twenty years have happened in developing countries. Thus, the poor nations—mostly traditional societies—would seem to be suffering the most, while the industrially developed world (America, Europe, and the Soviet Union, which have polluted the earth most by disregarding the natural order) have escaped the brunt of these events. The idea of natural order, however, would seem to include an element of natural justice. Would you comment on the apparent contradiction?**

The world community is one. Prosperous countries are dependent upon the prosperity of the underdeveloped countries. If disasters occur in underdeveloped countries, prosperous societies also will be greatly affected. In fact, when underdeveloped countries are hurt, the eventual suffering in the prosperous countries is greater than when the situation is reversed.

When natural catastrophes hit one place, all places ultimately are affected. Furthermore, in the long historical view, we discover that when one place is hit and another is left unharmed, the comparatively untouched place will be hit sometime in the future or has already been hit in the past.

**So you're saying that there are invisible reverberations which extend worldwide?**

That's right. We have a tendency to think "this nation, that nation," "this area, that area." Because of this divided approach we may feel it is "unfair" when one country is hit and another is not hit. Instead we should strive to see always the whole picture.

**Conversely, would you also say that when one country benefits, then all benefit?**

Definitely.

**Do you see any connection between social disorder and natural catastrophes?**

There are two factors which cause natural catastrophes. The first is geological: continents change into oceans, oceans change into continents, mountains sink, valleys rise. This goes on continuously, regardless of whether humanity is living on the earth. However, there is another factor, the human catastrophe; social decomposition, war, biological decline, psychological degeneration, etc. These human patterns—especially via the means of present-day highly developed, huge industries—definitely influence and accelerate some natural catastrophes.

There are several theories concerning the human effect on the biosphere through atmospheric pollution, nuclear radiation, the lowering or raising of the earth's atmospheric temperature, and so forth. In these ways basic atmospheric changes arise. A change in atmospheric pressure, for example, affects the crust of the earth, which is the balance point between the mantle and the atmosphere. If major atmosphere change occurs, a natural imbalance arises and the crust changes in order to adjust to that. This adjustment sometimes takes the form of earthquakes. Such things are quite possible. But it is debatable to exactly what extent these things happen.

**One final, philosophical question: is there anything that stands outside of the order of the universe which you have been talking about?**

Unfortunately, nothing can stand outside the order of the universe—except the order of the universe itself. Our whole world, our very life, our civilization, our history; animals, plants, atoms, galaxies, stars; mental, psychological, and spiritual phenomena including the so-called world of spirits before or after death, each mechanism or reincarnation; each process of endless changes—all are governed by the order of the universe.

**So in fact there are no real "catastrophes."**

What appear as catastrophes in our limited view are actually adjustments toward harmony, and those changes are going on all the time.

# 9

# World Peace
# Through World Health

This summer my wife Aveline and I toured Europe, giving many seminars on the macrobiotic way of life. In Malaga we lectured in universities where over four hundred medical professors, doctors, and students attended. We also gave talks in Barcelona, Lisbon, Antwerp, Amsterdam, and Frankfurt.

Wherever we went, we found that people are rapidly degenerating from cancer, heart disease, mental illness, and other diseases. At the same time everyone is seeking solutions to the problems of social health, regional security, and world peace. I was repeatedly asked, "What do you think about the possibility of world war in the near future?" As the Polish crisis this autumn demonstrated, the invasion of European countries by the Soviet Union has become a distinct possibility. Although everyone is concerned with this threat, they still routinely attend to their day-to-day activities. When the subject of nuclear war comes up, Europeans immediately become very depressed and serious.

In Germany, it is especially tense. Both the Soviets and the Americans have military bases on German soil, and forces on both sides are mobilized to maximum levels. Neighboring countries are growing nervous as well. For example, in Switzerland many families have weapons and practice self-defense. Underground fallout shelters are now mandatory in all new houses. Switzerland is supposed to be a neutral nation, but the towns and villages are actively preparing for atomic war.

In Europe, then, World War III is not just an imaginary problem. After a review of recent events in Afghanistan, Korea, Southeast Asia, Iran, and the Middle East, I told our friends that I felt the possibility of

---

Originally published in December, 1980 (East West Journal Vol. 10 No. 12)

nuclear war in the near future is very great. I returned to America convinced that there is a 90 percent chance of global holocaust in the next decade. Because of the continuing biological degeneration of our health and the unceasing development and stockpiling of nuclear weapons, war will inevitably arise unless there is a drastic change in the consciousness of the entire world in the next ten years.

When the atomic bomb dropped on Hiroshima, the population of the region, including outlying villages and towns, was about one million people. About three hundred thousand were killed instantly by the blast. In training yards, whole regiments of soldiers going through drills were turned into ashes. People standing in front of concrete buildings disappeared in the flash of the explosion leaving only their shadows etched in the ruins. The frantic survivors searched for water along the banks of the many rivers in Hiroshima, but tens of thousands died from contamination. About 90 percent of the buildings in the city collapsed except a few which were constructed of steel and concrete. On the inside they were like skeletons, totally burned out. Even today, thirty-five years later, survivors continue to die of leukemia from the radioactive fallout of that explosion.

At the time that Hiroshima was bombed, I was nineteen years old. I had been drafted into the militia, and my unit was stationed on Kyushu Island guarding the local railroad station. When the news came of the attack upon Hiroshima, we could not understand what kind of bomb could have caused such misery and destruction. Our previous orders were to shoot back at enemy planes. But now we were instructed to take cover underground if any foreign planes were sighted.

Three days later, Nagasaki was bombed. Kyushu station was close by, and every day thousands and thousands of sick and dying people were brought in by rail. Survivors completely filled the trains, and some even clung to the tops and the sides of the cars. Many men, women, and children died while fleeing the city in this way, and a great number who arrived at our station were between life and death. In the destroyed city itself, all efforts to save people were useless because fallout was everywhere. For several days no outside rescue teams could enter the city. One by one the survivors continued to die, and we were powerless to alleviate their suffering.

Everyone should know how terrible nuclear weapons are and the unimaginable death and destruction that will result if they are ever employed again. After World War II many scientists who participated in the construction of the atomic bomb, including Einstein and Oppenheimer, saw the necessity for a world government. They realized that the human race could never survive another World War. But in the years since then the nuclear arms race has continued, the bombs have grown thousands of time more fatal, and today the very future of humanity is at stake. If there is a thermonuclear war between the United States and the Soviet Union, neither side will win. Radiation and fallout will eventually claim even those who have taken shelter underground. There is no safe place to hide and no effective means to survive.

If present events continue, nuclear war will come either by mistake, technical error, or by intention. What can we do to change this drift toward annihilation? I often think about this problem on my travels where I meet with people seeking to heal cancer, heart disease, or other serious illness. From the windows of the consultation rooms—whether in Lisbon, Tokyo, Buenos Aires, or Los Angeles—I look up at the same blue sky and white clouds and watch the different birds fly by, their wings glistening in the shining beams of the sun. Even with the threat of universal destruction hanging over us, I realize how wondrous and beautiful our planet still is, moving in the space of the universe, following an endless spiral of motion and energy.

Nature is always realizing harmony and making balance. The sun, the moon, and the seasons cycle in perfect order. Yet within this wonderful harmony, humanity is suffering from a plague of degenerative diseases and trembling on the brink of war. Why is humanity suffering from internal and external disease and chaos?

Pollution, crime, and the threat of war mirror the condition of our own internal health. Those who can solve the problem of illness are really those who can solve the problem of war. Those who cannot solve the problem of illness cannot solve the problem of war. In order to discover the underlying cause of sickness and war, we have to recall our place in the universe as human beings. Instead of looking at the whole, the modern mind divides life into fragments. We see the human body as a system of biological functions and chemical interactions to be dissected and analyzed under a microscope rather than as a dynamic organism totally interdependent with its environment. All aspects of human life are governed by the natural order of this planet. In turn, our planet is governed by the order of the solar system. Beyond that there is the influence of the Milky Way of which we are a tiny part, and further out the infinite universe. In other words, all human affairs (including happiness and unhappiness, sickness and health, comfort and difficulty, birth and death) are manifestations of the order of the universe.

Universal laws govern human affairs just as they regulate celestial movements and the motions of subatomic particles. When we are in harmony with these laws, health, well-being, and peace naturally follow. When we fail to maintain equilibrium, physical, psychological, and spiritual disorder results.

As human beings, we relate to the natural environment in three major ways. First, we adjust to the physical and biological environment through the foods we eat. Secondly, we maintain balance with the gaseous environment through the way we breathe. Thirdly, we interact with the vibrational environment, the invisible world of electromagnetic radiation, through thoughts and images we receive and give out.

If eating, breathing, and thinking are in harmony with the environment, individual health and social well-being naturally follow. Hence, all traditional cultures devised methods to achieve and maintain harmony, control breathing, and perfect thinking in the form of prayer, chanting, meditation, and various other exercises. However, eating is the most fundamental interchange between the environment and human beings, and eating properly was always recognized as the foundation of the other two measures.

Today food is still the key to solving both problems of sickness and war. In the twentieth century various political leaders, scientists, reformers, and spiritual advisers have advanced proposals for community harmony and world peace. These proposed solutions include agreements and treaties among nations, United Nations conferences, congressional and parliamentary resolutions, citizens' campaigns for disarmament, efforts to control nuclear power, negotiations to limit weapons of mass destruction, international development and social welfare systems to lessen tension and provide security, and various religious, educational, and psychological attempts to change our way of thinking. However, all of these endeavors have failed to achieve peace because they have overlooked the underlying determinant in our life: the physical food that creates the cells of our bodies and brains.

In history nearly all cultures paid primary attention to agriculture and ways of eating in harmony with nature and the larger cosmos. Traditional religions, including Judaism, Catholicism, Islam, Buddhism, Taoism, and Shinto, in the past followed dietary guidelines and doctrines in order to realize maximum physical, psychological, and spiritual well-being. The modern world has forgotten how to achieve individual and social harmony through the use of daily food.

All past cultures knew whole grains to be the staff of life. For example, in the Far East the word for peace—*wa*—is formed from the ideograms for *cereal grain* and *mouth*. By putting grains into our mouths, we naturally become peaceful. However, in modern times, whole grains have become almost unobtainable in the industrialized world. Only in the past few years have we begun to rediscover the underlying connection between the foods we eat. The Senate's 1977 report on *Dietary Goals* and the Surgeon General's 1979 report on national health confirm what traditional societies have always known: whole grains and vegetables create healthy individuals and a healthy society, while a diet heavy in meat, dairy foods, refined flour, sugar, and chemicalized foods results in serious illness, including destructive behavior.

The road back to health and the achievement of peace begins with a return to organic and natural methods of agriculture and food processing, and the daily consumption of whole foods. A family which has suffered cardiovascular disorders, cancer, diabetes, or other degenerative diseases is a microcosm of a society suffering from repeated conflicts and battles, depressions, and war. In both cases, the cure is the same: the return to a sane way of eating.

In the temperate climates of the world, including the United States, the Soviet Union, China, Europe, and Japan, the standard macrobiotic diet is:

1.  50 to 60 percent whole cereal grains such as organic brown rice, whole wheat, barley, rye, corn, oats, and buckwheat;
2.  25 to 30 percent vegetables, locally and seasonally grown, including a small amount of seaweed and algae;
3.  5 to 10 percent beans;
4.  5 to 10 percent soup, especially miso or vegetable-based soup;
5.  occasional fruit, locally and seasonally grown;
6.  occasional animal food, especially white-meat fish rather than meat or poultry;
7.  natural water (neither chemically treated nor distilled) and natural grain or herb beverages (with no fragrant, stimulant, or aromatic effects).

Most of these foods should be cooked in order to facilitate complete digestion, though smaller portions of vegetables and fruits may be consumed raw.

If this dietary pattern were widely implemented, allowing for modifications to accommodate changing personal and environmental needs, world health would begin to improve immediately. Social and cultural stability—and eventually world peace—would follow. Such a diet would also contribute to the ecology and economies of the world, with the following savings:

1.  Greater efficiency in the utilization of land since grain would go directly to human beings rather than to cattle.
2.  Energy savings from reduced processing and packaging of foods and independence from chemical, oil-based fertilizers. The consumption of locally grown food would cut back substantially on food imported long distances and from different climates, thus reducing transportation costs.
3.  Lowered food costs as a whole for each family and country.
4.  Reduced medical and social welfare expenses as a natural result of improved health.
5.  Increased employment, productivity, and efficiency as the health of workers and management improves.

Social stability will return as understanding, adaptability, and flexibility increase. Violence and crime and all their attendant social costs also will begin to fall and level off.

It may appear that this biological process of elevating humanity through proper diet would be too slow and gradual to have any impact on the critical world situation. But we must realize that so far all other solutions, however well-meaning, have failed to slow down or reverse the nuclear arms race. If diet is ignored, world peace will remain an illusory and elusive goal. Only if we are physically and mentally healthy shall we have the strength, vitality, and will to obtain our goal. For this correct food is essential.

Today's leaders and most of the population of the world are so sick that they cannot envision peaceful settlements to our present conflicts. Without a vision of a peaceful world, there can only be war. Intuitively we know that we cannot go on creating nuclear weapons indefinitely before they are used in war.

Each day we materialize our vision of the future. Every morning each of us awakes at a certain hour and keeps certain appointments that are important to us. We have a vision of doing certain things, and we materialize parts of that vision. In this way we are constantly creating the day-to-day world by materializing our vision of life.

Why do some people see war in the future while others see peace? Why are some people successful in achieving their vision, while others are too weak to materialize what they would like the future to be? As we have seen, our vision of life is largely the result of the food which our mothers ate during pregnancy and the food which we eat every day. This food gives rise to a certain type of vision—violent for some, peaceful for others—and also makes us either strong enough to materialize our dream or too weak to accomplish things in life.

Those who are sick can only see a sick vision of the future. The vision of those who are perpetuating the arms race is a destructive vision. We are now witnessing the materialization of that vision. Due to their own poor health, many leaders, as well as many ordinary people, can only see the destruction of the entire world.

As individual families around the world become healthier through macrobiotics, however, peaceful visions of the future will spread. Families will begin to meet in assemblies or in congresses to support and encourage one another beyond any differences in belief, race, age, sex, or economic class. Regardless of their numerical size, these first families will constitute the sprout of a giant tree which will blossom centuries later when a peaceful world is fully realized.

The guiding spirit of that new era will be familial love, respect, and care. All aspects of human life will be affected, including religious and philosophical thought, scientific and technological development, economic and material distribution, and artistic and aesthetic expression. All will realize their common origin and ancestors and have a shared dream of the future. Elders will extend their love and care toward the younger generation. The young will respect and care for the elders. Man and woman will genuinely love, respect, and care for each other. Children and parents will live together in harmony. Families will respect and care for their community, nature and the environment, and the universe as a whole.

Outlines of that peaceful era are already becoming visible:

1. The political system will be replaced by a world council of elders composed of the most healthy, wise, and peaceful men and women.

Political systems shall change their orientation from governing, ruling, controlling, and regulating people into educational and service functions.

2.  The economic system will combine a respect for regional self-sufficiency (especially in agriculture, clothing, and housing) with world interdependency (especially in technology, communications, and engineering). Basic industries will be run more collectively, while secondary enterprises and small businesses will be operated along lines of free enterprise.

3.  The military system will be abolished and all weapons destroyed. Police systems shall be concerned less with law enforcement than with guarding and guiding physically and psychologically disabled people.

4.  The criminal reform system shall emphasize health care rather than punishment. It shall nourish offenders with proper food and ideas until their health is restored.

5.  The medical system shall emphasize prevention rather than cure, especially through dietary education. Medical treatments will be available on a small scale for critical conditions or emergencies.

6.  Artistic and literary expressions shall be respected, whether theoretical or practical, spiritual or materialistic, personal or social. Free expression is an essential part of a healthy and peaceful world.

7.  The educational system shall encourage self-reliance rather than received ideas or abstract information.

In the future world, research and discoveries shall confirm the invincible, permanent, immortal, and universal order of the universe. In daily life everyone will realize the practical unity of science and religion, philosophy and art, agriculture and spiritual development. The future world belongs to those who know the relationship between health and peace and who understand humanity's place in the world, the solar system, and the galaxy. The universe is our endless home. Our common dream is to realize health and happiness on earth together. For those people who presently are ill or face violence, it is imperative to begin macrobiotics immediately in order to survive this period of transition. For those who are already macrobiotic, it is not enough to eat well. At this time they must go out into the community and actively work to create harmony and build a world family. Together we can end the threat of nuclear war and build one peaceful world.

# III

# EDUCATION

# 10

# Family Roots: Do You Know Who Your Great-Grandparents Were?

Families fall into two general types: horizontal or vertical. Horizontal families center on the relationship between husband and wife, whereas vertical families stress the continuity between ancestors and descendants. The vertical is the more traditional form, and the horizontal is a relatively modern phenomenon.

A more horizontal structure is typical of most families today in the United States. In this structure, the husband and wife form a more or less independent unit. When the children have grown up, they in turn go out to establish their own relatively independent unit. Of course, some friendly, social relations may exist between the families of brothers and sisters, but the relationships do not extend very deeply.

This horizontal pattern is typical of modern industrialized nations, where the main question in life tends to be the individual's means of earning a living. That emphasis dates from about the seventeenth century, at the dawn of the industrial age. As a result of changes in the economic and social structure of society which first appeared around that time, people nowadays generally will select their residence according to where work is available; the resulting mobility operates as a disintegrating factor on the ties between brothers, sisters, and other relatives. As those bonds weaken, the traditions uniting family members gradually disappear; thus, very few people today know much about their great-grandparents or even grandparents. In comparison to the memory span of a vertical family extending over countless generations of ancestors, the lifespan of any one horizontal family is very short, normally including only two or, at most, three generations.

---

Originally published in March, 1978 (East West Journal Vol. 8 No. 3)

Even today the vertical form is still the general rule in the Orient—e.g. China, India, Indonesia, Japan, and Southeast Asia. It is characterized by unity among the generations which also serves to unite siblings strongly, even after marriage. The unity of the vertical family is maintained by three factors: dietary, spiritual, and practical.

Dietary unity means that the family has a typical style of cooking which is passed on from mother to daughter and daughter-in-law. Since we are what we eat, the generations of such families tend to resemble each other in physique and personality. Their characteristic way of eating is maintained by the custom of a bride's coming to live with the groom's parents for two or three months before the wedding in order to learn the family's typical cooking methods. After she has learned how to carry on the family's traditional diet, the new couple is free to set up a household on their own.

This physiological unity is reinforced by a spiritual practice emphasizing reverence for ancestors. A quiet room is normally set aside in the main home of the extended family, where some type of shrine, no matter how simple, is dedicated to the spirits of deceased family members. The head of the house meditates or prays there every morning and evening. Each branch of the family has a miniature of this shrine in its house, and members of the branch families pay their respects to it daily. Even if some of the branch families live far away, the whole clan gathers every year or so for a reunion. These celebrations normally include some kind of memorial ceremony or acknowledgment of the ancestors.

The biological and spiritual unity is further cemented by a set of shared norms, which particularly apply when choosing marriage partners. These norms include agreed-upon standards of behavior, such as honesty, ethical business practices, the enjoyment of simple pleasures, etc. The Mosaic code, which unified all the Jewish tribes, is an example of that approach embodied within the Western tradition and uniting the Jewish people over their long history.

In the vertical family, parents and often grandparents initiate children into the family's ethical heritage by praising or pointing out the inadequacy of the children's behavior specifically in terms of that code and its precedents. If one member of a vertical family falls upon hard times or gets into trouble, the older members assemble for a family counsel. If a particular individual, for example, is put in jail for some crime, they decide whether to work for his release and how to go about that or perhaps even to let him remain in jail as a justified lesson. Conversely, if one family member receives some outstanding honor, the whole family feels proud and throws a big celebration party.

In the vertical family, selection of a spouse involves everyone's participation and approval, because the new couple will be carrying on the traditions of a much larger unit than itself. In forming a horizontal family, the young couple may ask for their parents' opinions, but in most cases the real decision has already been made. To a certain extent, members of a horizontal family may share some spiritual unity through their religion, but that also tends to be a minor factor in their marriage. As for dietary unity, it has been almost completely lost through the modern massive changeover to commercially manufactured food, which is prepared in a uniform manner with of course no thought for variation between families.

Both the horizontal and the vertical patterns have their advantages and disadvantages. However, in my opinion excessive stress in recent times has been placed on the advantages of the horizontal family and the disadvantages of the vertical family. It is worth keeping in mind that, although the preservation of a vertical structure involves certain difficulties, those very obstacles can be taken as challenges; they expand the game of life to include the context of many generations spanning greater reaches of time than are dealt with by horizontal families mutually isolated over geographical space.

For anyone who is interested in restoring the unity of his or her vertical family, I would suggest beginning in the following manner.

First, learn how to select, prepare, and serve foods in a way that will ensure your family's health, and pass this knowledge on to everyone in your family circle who is interested. Second, keep in touch with all members of your family through regular correspondence, calls, and visits, particularly on traditional holidays. When you visit your parents or brothers and sisters, offer to cook a natural dish for them—but if they are not interested do *not* insult them by refusing to eat their food; enjoy in moderation what they offer you and show them your loving spirit. Third, set aside a regular time to remember your ancestors with gratitude. Fourth, start to write a history of your family.

Where did your parents, grandparents and ancestors come from? What kinds of things did they do? What kind of people were they? Try to find out their places of birth and death and all their children's names.

Then give copies of this record to your own children, advising them to extend it further. That way you can rekindle the flame of your traditional family and pass it on to the future generations.

# 11

## Helping Children Learn

**Do you have any particular method that you would recommend for helping a child learn to talk?**

Children begin to talk in a very natural way, making their own sounds, coming out with their own words. Let them speak frequently in their own way. You need not teach them any definite words until they are about three or four months old. Then you can gradually introduce adult words, repeating them very slowly. Children tend to repeat words many times, but they do that only because the parents talk too rapidly for them to grasp the word at first hearing. An adult's way of speaking is quicker than that of infants because the lengths of children's brain waves are appreciably longer than those of adults. As we grow up, the brain waves become shorter. Therefore when talking to children, adults should speak more slowly than normal; then children can understand them easily and will need to repeat words only once or twice, instead of many times. If you speak slowly, children will understand adult words very easily. The same principle should be applied whenever you read stories to children. If you read the story slowly, after one or two times the children will understand and even memorize it very easily.

When you write letters or numbers for them, use a larger size so that their brains, which deal more easily with larger images, can grasp the forms more readily. In my opinion many children who have problems learning to speak have been incorrectly designated as mentally retarded, when in fact they have simply been taught at too rapid a tempo and with letters and numbers that are too small for them to understand readily.

---

Originally published in July, 1977 (East West Journal Vol. 7 No. 7)

Because they have been taught at adult speed and with adult sizes of letters and objects, they cannot catch up. By always proceeding slowly and using larger sizes of letters and objects, we can ensure that by the age of five our children can have a command of many adult expressions.

At the same time that mental development is proceeding, children are also developing physically. Mental development follows upon the physical development. So the child should be active in both play and learning. Adults should not interfere with the child's physical development. For example, if parents are overprotective or frequently pick up a child who is just learning to crawl or walk, the child's physical and therefore mental development will be impaired. During the embryonic period, before birth, a baby develops through all the stages of biological evolution at the rate of about 10 million years per day, totalling about three billion years of biological evolution before birth. About one-and-a-half years after birth babies can stand up straight, walk, and talk. This period corresponds to about 400 million years of human evolution. That breaks down to about 700 to 800 years of biological evolution per minute for the child's first one-and-a-half years of life. If a parent picks up a child for one minute, interrupting his or her crawling or walking, that means interfering with about 700 to 800 years of biological development.

Crawling is very important to a baby, because the muscles and joints are developed and strengthened through this vigorous activity. Concommitant with this activity children are also developing their brains and power of sensory judgment. Only after babies have become proficient at one stage, can they proceed normally to the next stage of physical and mental development. Therefore it is crucial for the child to be active and develop at his or her own pace and not be interrupted by an overprotective parent.

### How would you explain children's widely differing speeds of development?

That large variation is due to the different forms of nutrition that children ingest to build their bodies. We should not give children food that will make them mature too quickly. A diet containing dairy food, for example, will make children grow faster physically, but they will remain mentally relatively less developed, because their mental growth cannot keep up with the abnormally stimulated physical growth. Human beings should be about one year old before standing up, even one-and-a-half years is still all right. A baby who grows teeth very early or who shows other signs of maturing extremely early, is suffering from an imbalanced diet, usually an alarmingly high percentage of animal protein. Protein is an essential factor for growth, but taken in excess it speeds up development beyond a healthy, natural rate. Animal food should constitute at most about one-eighth, or 15 percent, of the human diet. Of course, you don't need to give children any animal food at all: e.g., red meat, poultry, eggs, fish, milk, cheese, etc. They can grow very well obtaining all the protein they need for growth from a totally vegetarian diet.

On the other hand, some children develop very slowly. Babies who aren't walking by the time they are almost two years old are usually suffering from one of two factors: excess salt in their diet or not enough fresh vegetables. Because of its constrictive power physiologically, too much salt prevents a baby from expanding and growing normally. Fresh vegetables, on the other hand, are essential because of their expansive effects physiologically. In the case of many modern children who eat foods containing sugar, chemicals, or a large amount of fruit (e.g. daily orange juice), slow development could indicate another kind of weakness: mental retardation caused by the harmful effects of these foods on the nervous system. In general, therefore, slow development is caused by three main factors: too much yang (over-contractive foods such as salt), too much yin (such as sugar, chemicals, or excessive fruit), or too much interference on the part of the parents.

### Earlier you called the sounds babies make, which we consider nonsense syllables, a language. What is that language?

The language of babies is a highly symbolic one. When a baby says one word, it includes many meanings. Children have a full range of concepts but can't formulate them in precise detail. The scope of babies' concepts is actually as broad as adults', but their concepts are not expressed in such analytical detail. The adult mentality gives clarity and precision to each part of that generalized understanding. An adult may use about ten thousand words to express concepts for which a child uses only about twenty. During the early period of mental development, if children are bombarded with too many fragmentary adult concepts, they can't develop their innate, intuitive understanding. We should let children talk to themselves, to dogs, flowers, anything, in their own language. Then gradually the more detailed expression of adult society will emerge.

**When children begin school, the first requirement is vaccination. Many of our readers, however, object to that. What advice would you offer on this question?**

The idea behind immunizations is to create a mild sickness artificially so that the body will develop a resistance to any later appearance of the same sickness. But why are some peole susceptible to an illness which does not affect others? Their resistance is low, because their daily way of life, especially their daily way of eating, is unhealthy. If our way of eating and way of life are healthy, we do not get sick. There is no reason to make someone artificially sick. By doing that, a resistance is created to certain diseases, but at the same time, some other aspects of the growing process is impaired, since the natural developmental abilities are being used up in resisting and battling that artificially induced sickness.

We should avoid vaccinations as far as possible. The idea of using vaccinations is based on a misconception of the natural order: modern people think that some invading, foreign element, such as a bacteria or virus, is the cause of illness; so they plan a counterattack through artificial immunizations. But germs are not ultimately the cause of illness; they are merely the agent by which we become aware of our unhealthy condition. The real cause is the unhealthy quality of our blood, due to an unhealthy way of eating that predisposes the individual to illness. Artificial treatments such as immunizations are attempts to compensate for an already existing low level of vitality.

Many governments require immunizations; however, it is sometimes possible to maneuver around that legal formality. For example, in France, Belgium, and a few other countries there is now a trend to make vaccinations not compulsory but simply available to those who want them. This civil movement is becoming more widespread now. I hope that eventually this country, too, will allow people freedom of choice on the question of medical procedures such as immunizations. If we are eating poorly, there is definitely a need for these medications. If the family cannot nourish children properly with healthy food, then they may feel some justifiable fear and decide to have their children vaccinated. However, that process of vaccination may be the seed of some serious physical or mental problems later on. The whole point of health care is to eat properly and live in harmony with the laws of nature.

## Would you be more specific about what you mean when you say that our diet should be in harmony with the laws of nature?

Human beings are able to eat foods from almost the entire biological world. From conception to birth we nourish ourselves from the essence of the animal world—that is, our mother's bloodstream. After we are born, we continue to be nourished from our mother's blood in the form of mother's milk, which is a less concentrated animal food than blood itself. When we can stand erect we have reached the stage of evolution of human beings. At that time we start to eat foods from the whole spectrum of the vegetable kingdom. We graduate from animal-food eating and begin eating from the vegetable kingdom as our biological ancestors did in the evolutionary process.

Grains evolved on earth at the same time as *Homo sapiens*. Since they made possible the evolution of human beings as a species, cereal grains form the main part of our diet as the "staff of life," with vegetables and small amounts of other food as side dishes. This general pattern is what I mean by eating in harmony with the laws of nature.

## What is the purpose of education?

At the present time the main purpose of education is to make the child develop into a socially adapted and useful person: i.e., someone who will eventually make a contribution to the prosperity of society by earning a living, working in some organizations, perhaps pursuing an intellectual career, etc. Certainly these activities have some merit, but they form only a part of life. Modern education neglects many essential areas of existence.

The primary purpose of education is to help children become healthy, happy, and strong as human beings, not only as social persons. In order to accomplish that, we need to develop their understanding of why they came here, why they were born, what their largest goals are, and how to maintain their health and happiness while on this earth. That is the essential kind of human intelligence, sometimes called common sense, which education should foster as its primary goal. Second come the technical problems involved in preserving health, developing our powers of judgment, behaving properly in various situations, and dealing correctly with other people. Third comes the kind of social relations that modern education handles, such as what kind of technical service can be performed as an adult. So modern education alone is not enough. Prior to that kind of education, we need a broad basic education as human beings.

In grammar school all children should learn to take basic care of themselves. Those elementary skills include maintaining their health, selecting and preparing their daily food, taking care of their clothes, knowing how to construct simple shelters and how to grow food; they should also be introduced to a basic awareness of what our place is within the natural world, including the relationship of our earth to the surrounding universe. All these matters of basic common sense should be established in grammar school.

In high school this basic education should be continued, but new subjects can be introduced, such as human relationships, for example, learning how to show respect for elders, acting in a loving way to younger people, and generally dealing with people in society. High-school students should also study history, geography, the social and natural sciences, and other academic subjects.

Unlike children subjected to modern education, which is completely fragmented, because it has no underlying principle that works in all areas, children should be learning the universal principle of balance, or yin and yang, from the very start of grammar school through all of high school and on through college. This principle should inform all aspects of their education: e.g., it can be used in studying physics, chemistry, health, cooking, social sciences, etc. College should involve some kind of original creation using yin and yang. Students at that stage should discover or invent something on their own. College-level studies can be completed by the age of seventeen or eighteen. After that, young people can explore whatever they want in order to gain social experience. They can begin any kind of independent research or travel for adventure.

**The way you described children learning about food and clothing during the grammar school years sounds like education in any traditional culture living close to nature. How would you advise us, as modern Westerners, to help our children develop a similar understanding even though we live in a modern city?**

A major part of early education should be children's participation in productive family activities. Teach them basic cooking. Let them help with sewing, cooking, baking, etc. Take them on a tour through a small factory so they can see how clothes are made. The same thing applies to carpentry, gardening, and other household skills.

**The school that you have been describing doesn't have much in common with today's schools. How can parents who disagree with the current educational system handle the differences between the ideology taught in today's schools and the philosophy by which they live in their own homes?**

If we don't have our own schools yet, obviously our children must go to public school or private school, but then home education becomes even more important. Use every opportunity to teach your children outside of school about life, including the basic skills I mentioned. Parents should also explain to their children the order of nature, in terms of yin and yang, and help them develop, through their own observations, a way of seeing the complementary relationships in nature and between people.

**In many cases children are being taught one set of values at home—how to eat in harmony with nature, how to behave toward others in a non-competitive way—and a quite different point of view in school. How can we help them to make sound judgments on their own between these two varying ideologies?**

Never tell children what not to do; don't say, for example, "You shouldn't eat school lunches" or "You should not believe what the teacher says about nutrition," etc. Instead, let the children select for themselves and experience what they want. Now, when they have some experience, there is always a result. When that result appears, for example, if children eat ice cream or candy and later don't feel well, then ask them, "Why do you feel bad today? What do you think is the cause? Did you eat some ice cream or candy?" That way the children will understand. So, first, their daily food at home should be very good. Second, children should be encouraged to understand all phenomenon as expressions of balance, or yin and yang. Third, parents can, at dinnertime, give children a question and let them figure it out themselves.

**Modern education seems to emphasize competitiveness. I remember how important grades were for me in school. How do you see the personal abilities that are sometimes overlooked in school or even at home?**

Nothing in this relative world stays the same; nothing is identical. Even in the case of twins of the same sex, the space occupied in the mother's womb and the time of delivery is different. Each fetus in the womb selects different qualities of food from the mother's blood. All people are different. No one is superior in all ways to other people.

Children are evaluated today in a very narrow scope. Some children have an excellent school record, but that is only one small part of the whole person. The standard used in present-day evaluations at school is very conceptual and one-sided. If children have a good mechanical memory, then they will be high scorers. But that kind of rote memory is only a very small part of human intelligence. Much more important are the children's insights, their broad understanding and clear powers of judgment. Those factors, however, do not show up on school records. Most important of all is their physical, mental, and spiritual health. That, again, doesn't appear on school records.

Some children go to school and get a D, while others may get an A, but the most important thing is which group was putting forth its best effort. The child's ability to try is most important, and the marks received are only of secondary importance. Parents should encourage their children to do their best at whatever they like to do. They should emphasize, "Do your best in school, in society, in whatever you like to do, and don't worry about competition. When you do your best in what you really want to do, that is the best."

Parents should give guidance on this point, because the school doesn't provide for it. You can totally erase any idea of competition. Many great world leaders had very low school records. Just encourage children to do their best, whether in school or at home. When they put forth their best effort, it doesn't matter whether their marks in school are the best or the worst—they have done wonderfully.

# 12

# Education For Freedom

I propose a school that teaches the unification of all antagonistic opposites. Those who pass through this school will be noticeable for their health, their ability to create order, and their high judgment. They will be the ones to bring about a world event of great magnitude which we are witnessing in our lifetimes, the reconciliation of East and West.

Let us consider a possible program for the education of our children which is divided into twelve levels, the students' ages corresponding at each level to the current system of education in the United States—that is, beginning around age six and ending around age eighteen. There are five basic areas of study:

1.  Nature (physics, chemistry, biology),
2.  Humanity and society,
3.  Creative skills (language, literature, art, and technology),
4.  Mathematics,
5.  Daily life (physical education and home economics).

In the first grade, children learn about the complementary opposites yin and yang as revealed in basic phenomena of nature: shapes, colors, tastes, movement. Instruction in the area of humanity and society is presented in combination with literature by reading them stories and fairy tales that also serve to develop the imagination. A sense of fellowship with all cultures is encouraged by singing songs from all over the world. Meditation is practiced at the start of each day in every grade. The alphabet and counting are repeatedly chanted aloud in unison, for

---

Originally published in September, 1978 (East West Journal Vol. 8 No. 9)

chanting improves circulation and develops physical keenness. The essential rudiments of social behavior—how to greet parents and elders, how to express gratitude and to apologize—are taught along with such practical skills as personal hygiene and keeping their school environment clean and orderly. It is important that children learn to create order from the beginning of their school experience. In each grade level, most classroom work is done in the morning, leaving the afternoons free for agricultural outings, sports events, etc. There should be ample time for outdoor play, as well as origami, painting, writing, drawing, and other creative activities. Students at this level begin to learn the use of various art media—pencils, crayons, water colors, oils, and black and white brush work—in the progressive order of difficulty, with the medium changing every second year. Also, at mealtime, they learn to chew their food well and to eat peacefully.

Children in the second grade study yin and yang in nature—directions, weight, temperature, polarity (plus and minus), etc., and in daily life—cold vesus hot baths, sweet versus salty toothpaste, eating from yang to yin at mealtimes. Teachers continue reading aloud to them, emphasizing fairy tales and imaginative literature.

In the third grade, students learn about yin and yang in the environment (for example, seasonal changes), in the human body (organs, bones, etc.), in their social surroundings (relationships among peers, elders, parents, siblings, students and teachers), and in creative skills, especially language and literature. Students are taught to read aloud—a practice to be continued in the higher grades, since this aids the development of clear speech and provides the same physical benefits as unison chanting. Again teachers read aloud to the students, but the selections are now chosen from the best writing of all cultures (the Bible, Confucius, etc.). The children grow their own vegetable garden and begin to make tools and instruments.

In the fourth grade, children study yin and yang in animals, plants, the cycles of the moon and winds, the development of life forms, basic classification, and in many other aspects of their environment. They begin a study of foreign languages which will continue throughout their school years. They learn to play the flute (the simplest instrument—the greatest skill), and study interior decorating and domestic skills like washing clothes and dishes.

Fifth graders study material yin and yang, the physics of temperature and pressure and states of change. Scale measurements and geometry are added to their mathematical studies. Their social studies extend to the community. Composition, grammar, and poetry are stressed. There is an emphasis on team sports and martial arts, as well as basic cooking—the preparation of bread, rice, and vegetables.

In the sixth grade, nature studies focus upon biological life. The social view expands to encompass the country as a whole, examining the inter-relationships of transportation, economic, and political systems.

From the seventh grade, at puberty, boys and girls begin to diverge in their studies, except in certain basic areas. However, the option is always open for them to study subjects in which they have a strong interest—girls can learn carpentry; boys, sewing, etc. In the seventh grade students learn about the non-material world of energy—the spirit. They study yin and yang as reflected in the dialectics of world history, in literature, and in composition. They begin making furniture, and learn other manual skills; the gardens they planted as third-graders now include grains as well as vegetables.

Students in the eighth grade are encouraged to express themselves creatively in sculpture, painting, poetry, and music. Working with black and white brush painting—the simplest, most difficult art medium—they are taught to strive towards the ultimate goal of art: to express the largest in the smallest, infinity in the infinitesimal, the highest art evoking the boundless void.

Ninth graders study yin and yang in the solar system, the galaxies, the universe; in the rise and fall of ancient civilizations; in such mechanical technologies as motors and power sources; and in domestic economics—savings, budgets, income management.

In the tenth grade, perhaps the most conceptual year of their education, students learn the laws of change as a whole; how to develop health, social peace, and justice; the motivations and origins of technology and politics. They are encouraged to begin to define their own individual dream, their own philosophy of life.

The last two years merge into a single course, designed as a transition into society. There are many directions a student might follow in these years: exchange programs with foreign students; the publishing of books, articles, poetry; art exhibits; work-study programs; farming; studies in domestic life—birth, child care, home medicine; meditation and philosophy; community planning; archaeology; wilderness expeditions; crafts of all kinds. Each student is given the opportunity to follow his or her own personal dream.

It should be evident from this outline, which points out only the salient features of the curriculum at each grade level, that we study all those subjects ordinarily taught in modern schools, plus many more.

In our system of education there are no tests and no grades. Individual students are evaluated according to the following criteria: Are they healthy? Are they creative? Are they orderly? Do they relate well to others?

Freedom requires self-discipline. Our aim is to develop this quality in each student. The way for the teacher to handle disruptive behavior is to apologize in front of the class for the misbehaving student. The teacher must assume responsibility for everything that happens in his or her classroom. This approach causes the disruptive student to feel remorseful and reestablishes a sense of unity in the class.

The teacher's responsibility also extends to mealtimes. A cafeteria-style arrangement is most suitable. It is the teacher's task to determine the special dietary needs of each pupil: some may need eggs or fish; some may need more or less salt. Meals for children should be cooked with a minimum of salt; salted condiments can be offered in the form of gomasio, tamari, etc. The teacher always eats with his or her students, sitting with different children each day so that he or she may observe their eating patterns and make recommendations.

The process of education is threefold: first, unification of mental, physical, and spiritual growth through proper eating in harmony with the natural order; second, discovery of one's own individual dream by exercising the imagination and recognizing that all of life is play; third, contemplation of the laws of change—the Order of the Universe—through intuition. The passive (yin) aspect of intuition is judgment; the active (yang) aspect is will. The quality of our intuition, of our judgment and will, and the spirit with which we approach life, depend ultimately upon the quality of the food we eat. When a person has developed sound intuition, a high level of judgment, and a strong will, that person is free.

The school should provide an atmosphere of fun and play. Teachers must be imaginative in their search for ways to present all subjects in this spirit. For example, sports can be used not only as physical education, but also as lessons in mathematics, measuring distance and time. Nature trips can be used for countless studies besides biology. Learning should be an adventure which students will desire to continue long after their formal schooling has ended.

# IV

# A NEW WORLD

# 13

# The Ancient World

Any advance in knowledge involves two steps: first we form a picture of the truth, and then we check that vision against the facts. Every great scientist has been a dreamer; imagination is not confined to artists alone. How, otherwise, could modern scientists have visualized a model of the atom? The intuitive image came first. In order to form an image of the ancient past or the distant future, our first step should be reading mythology and prophecies, historical novels and science fiction to pick up the imaginative clues which can then be compared with the factual evidence from scientific disciplines such as astronomy and archaeology.

Heinrich Schliemann, who founded modern archaeology on the principle that epic works like Homer or the Bible refer to historical events and are not the mere fancy which the pedants of his time considered them to be, offers a dramatic example of this method. He discovered the historic site of the Trojan War, recounted in Homer, by pursuing through many difficulties the inspiration of a childhood vision. Gerald Hawkins, who discovered Stonehenge's function as an astronomical observatory, was similiarly impelled on his revolutionary path by the strenth of his imagination. His great imaginative leap was in forming the unsettling idea that people thousands of years ago were highly intelligent and capable of surveying the heavens mathematically. The second stage of that discovery—checking his intuition by feeding data on the position of the huge pillars at Stonehenge into a modern computer—was of course necessary, for theories that cannot be correlated with evidence remain empty speculations.

Originally published in February, 1974 (East West Journal Vol. 4 No. 2)

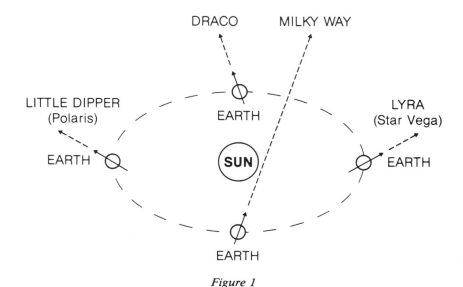

*Figure 1*

Dream and fact must go together, but in order to evaluate their coordination we need a unifying principle that is broad and flexible enough to embrace the worlds both of mind and of matter, imaginative vision and scientific data. The essays in this book are examples of how that unifying principle called yin and yang, balance, or complementarity, can be applied to any domain.

As the earth spins around the sun, it slowly wobbles like a top, with its north-south axis pointing first in one direction, then in the other, making one complete wobble every 25,800 years. That roughly 26,000-year wobbling motion of the earth's axis traces a circle across the sky, with first one northern constellation and then another serving as the pole star (see Figure 1). In order to understand the character of the ancient, and the future worlds, we must examine the phases in this large cycle of 25,800 years which governs the precession of the equinoxes.

In 2102 A.D., the earth's north-south axis will point almost directly at Polaris in the Little Dipper. About 13,000 years ago, half-way back on this cycle, the pole star was Vega in the constellation of Lyra, the Harp. In another 13,000 years Vega again will be the pole star, and before that comes about, the earth's north-south axis will be oriented toward the Milky Way—roughly 6500 years from now (see Figure 2).

Stonehenge has taught us that the ancients had a very keen appreciation for astronomical cycles. Evidence for a highly sophisticated

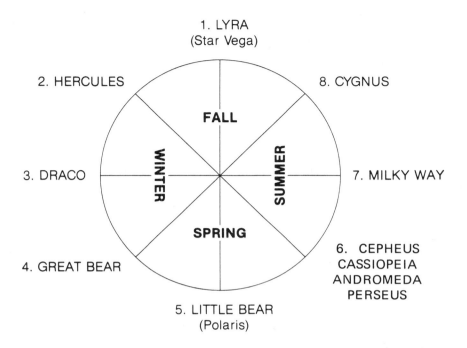

1. LYRA
(Star Vega)

2. HERCULES

8. CYGNUS

FALL

WINTER

SUMMER

3. DRACO

7. MILKY WAY

SPRING

4. GREAT BEAR

6. CEPHEUS
CASSIOPEIA
ANDROMEDA
PERSEUS

5. LITTLE BEAR
(Polaris)

*Figure 2*

awareness of the 26,000-year cycle among people predating even the builders of Stonehenge comes to us from the evidence of mythology around the world. In the Western tradition this particular cycle appears in a cluster of myths concerning various circumpolar constellations in the northern sky.

Everyone must have been struck at least once by the strange fact that the constellations don't resemble, except in a seemingly quite arbitrary way, the figures which they are supposed to represent. The constellation of Cassiopeia, for example, looks much more like the letter 'W' than the princess in Greek mythology whose name it bears. If those five stars are going to be grouped as one form, why not call them simply Two Valleys, or Three Mountains?

The solution to this riddle is that the circle of circumpolar constellations as a whole tell a story, the voyage of human civilizations through the stages of the 26,000-year cycle. The ancients used the patterns of stars in the night sky as we use printed books, movies, or television—as a medium for preserving and conveying information. Most people are

familiar with such a celestial type of medium in the twelve signs of the
Zodiac, which describe in a kind of symbolic shorthand the sequence of
natural change over one year. Let us now study a cycle of eight constellations which circle the central part of the sky almost directly overhead and
cover the cycle of 26,000 years.

That great cycle falls into two halves, which can be called light and
darkness, or the Time of Paradise and the Time of Struggle. It can be
divided further into four seasons: first, summer, or the peak of light; next
fall; then, winter, or the depth of darkness; and finally, spring. Transi-
tional stages of four more constellations between these four points make a
total of eight constellations in the cycle (see Figure 2).

These eight stages of transformation are represented in the eight
trigrams of Fu Hsi, which form the basis of the *I Ching* or "Book of
Changes." For those unacquainted with that fundamentally binary
Chinese system, we will use the more complicated but more readily
familiar Western system of eight constellations described in Greek
mythology and the Judaeo-Christian tradition (see Figure 3).

1.  Let's begin in the autumn of this cycle with Vega (whose name is an
    Arabic word meaning "fall"). It is in the constellation of the Harp,
    linked with the musician Orpheus, who descended to the dark
    underworld searching for his bride Euridice. Vega is not, of course, a
    "falling" or "shooting" star; its otherwise inexplicable name refers
    to the mythological "fall from Paradise," marking the time roughly
    13,000 years ago when the world was engulfed in the great Flood,
    due to an axis shift, recounted in most mythologies of the world and
    best known to us in the Old Testament story of Noah.

2.  After the great destruction by water under Vega, an enormous task
    of reconstruction had to be undertaken, and the next constellation
    after Vega is Hercules, the Greek hero famous for the performance
    of an almost endless list of extremely difficult tasks, mainly reclama-
    tion projects and killing or capturing savage beasts. Our ancestors
    10,000 years ago struggling to rebuild a world shattered by The
    Flood must have been occupied in just such labors.

3.  The entire left side of the circle covering the period from 12,000 years
    ago to the present is dominated by Draco, the Dragon, the serpent of
    Biblical tradition, associated with the expulsion from the Garden of
    Eden. A star in the tail of Draco, one-quarter of the way around the
    circle, is the pole star the furthest removed on the cycle from the

Milky Way. Draco rules the deepest darkness in which mankind was submerged 6000 years ago preceeding the dawn of recorded civilization around 4000 B.C.

4. Next on the cycle, after Draco, comes the Great Bear. The story of the Greek hero Ulysses, whose wanderings over the Mediterranean are told in the Odyssey, was rooted in an ancient myth referring to a great bear hibernating in the winter and then re-emerging in the spring. His epic refers to the period about 4,000 years ago when civilization began to spread out from established centers and explored the world again. Ulysses, the patron saint of Western Man the Explorer, struggles past great obstacles and temptations to return to his wife Penelope, the spinner (whom we recognize in the Chinese name for Vega, the "Spinning Maid," who tries to rejoin her lover across the bridge of the Milky Way).

5. After the Great Bear comes the Little Bear, the "Second Beast" of Revelations, who rules the present era of fire (opposite the water deluge that occurred under Vega). The universally prophecied "destruction by fire" need not be sudden in the form of a nuclear holocaust, as so many imagine, but may be gradual and in fact already upon us in the form of catastrophic industrial pollution of both the external and internal environment.

6. The following stage takes us to Cepheus and Cassiopeia, the father and mother of Andromeda, chained to a rock by her parents as a sacrifice to the Dragon but rescued by the hereo Perseus. This incident symbolizes the loosening of the stringent shackles of a necessarily artificial and oppressively organized civilization which ruled during the 12,000-year domination of the Dragon in the dark half of the cycle; during that difficult period of scarcity cooperation for productivity had to be enforced by strongly centralizing social forces.

7. After that configuration, we reach the Milky Way cluster of light, when the plane of our galaxy spreads directly overhead with all the stars encircling that shining, heavenly field. This configuration prevailed approximately 19,000 years ago and will again cover the northern sky roughly 6000 years from now.

8. After the Milky Way, Cygnus (the dying swan whose song before her death is associated with great beauty and its plaintive end) brings us back to Vega in the harp of Orpheus. Cygnus signifies the time of decadence that follows the Golden Age of the Milky Way, and it precedes the Fall marked by Vega.

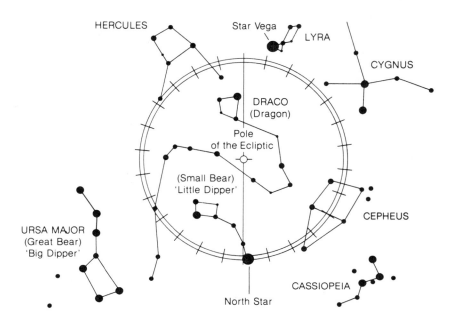

*Figure 3*

Traces of the same myth cluster around the figure of Hyperborean Apollo, who travels in his swan chariot to the mysterious realm whose inhabitants know neither sickness and old age, nor toils and warfare and live to great ages having spent most of their time dancing, making music, and feasting with crowns of bay leaves on their heads. It lies beyond (Hyper) the coldness of the North Wind (Boreas). Professor Cook in his volume *Zeus* shows that the path to the Hyperboreans was conceived of mythologically as the Milky Way.

Those interested can trace the same story in the Book of Revelations, with the clues that Babylon stands for the present era, and the "Woman clothes with the sun and the moon" is Vega situated between two bright stars. Her "child" is Hercules—who slaughtered a serpent in his crib. The "Great Beast from the Seas" corresponds to Ulysses the Mariner—i.e. the Great Bear.

The global distribution of these images represents the experience of the whole human race over a vast stretch of time. In the dark period under the Dragon, people struggled up from barbarism by organizing civilizations of ever greater extent and complexity. These artificial means to consolidate human efforts through institutions—such as the national state, official religions, massive technology, complex legal systems, etc.—were necessary for survival during the difficult period of reconstruction. The great weapon in that struggle was fire used in metallurgy, which now reaches the pinnacle of its development in modern industry.

The light half of the cycle, the Ancient World that was swept away in Noah's flood, is the realm described, for example, in the medieval romance of Sir Orpheo, where Orpheus finds his wife in a magical subterranean landscape.

> All that land was ever light
> For when it should be dark and night
> The rich stones light gunn *[gave off]*
> As bright as doth at noon the sun.

Let us now turn from an examination of the mythology surrounding this 26,000-year cycle to study the mechanism of its effects upon life on earth.

The sequence of changing light and darkness results from the distance across the sky which separates the Milky Way Galaxy from whatever constellation serves as the pole star at any particular time: Perseus and the Swan are not so far removed from the Milky Way, Vega and the Little Bear are the balancing points half-way toward the extreme point of separation; Hercules and Ulysses are further removed; the Dragon, or serpent, is the furthest removed from the light area of the Milky Way.

In order to understand the significance of that varying distance, picture the earth rotating on its north-south axis as a spool of thread balanced on the rim of a saucer, which represents our Milky Way Galaxy (see Figure 4). When the core (north-south axis) of the spool is tilted askew, no longer parallel to the surface of the saucer, it offers less of a permeable channel for the energies that flow along the surface of the saucer in the mass of stars forming that galactic disc. When the axis of the spool, however, is aligned parallel to the plane of the saucer, it is directly traversed by that enormous flow of galactic current. Thus, when the earth's axis points directly through the Milky Way we receive much more energy radiation than we do when the earth's axis points away from the Milky Way.

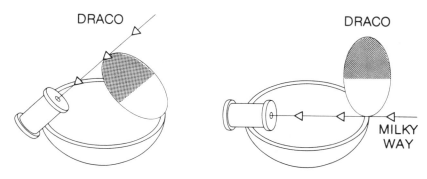

*Figure 4*

Next we must see how celestial influences such as the galactic current of energy radiation affect life forms on earth. The details of that process appear in our forthcoming article on acupuncture which explains the decisive importance for our physical, mental, and spiritual vitality of the energy channel which runs vertically through the center of the body. All the acupuncture meridians take their source from that internal meridian, or axis; they originate from it, like the ridges of a pumpkin curving out from the plant's central core.

When the earth is aligned with the plane of the galaxy, the great mass of stars clustered in that plane shed their influence directly down through the central, vertical (north-south) energy channel both of the planet and also of humanity as well as all other life forms on earth. Not only is the human brain much more active during that period, but all the botanical sources of our food are much more vigorous, requiring hardly any cultivation. This is the time of the Garden of Eden, or the Golden Age, which—to cite only one example—the Roman poet Virgil described as below:

"Now the last age has come as foretold by the sibyl of Cumae *[an ancient site of prophecy in southern Italy from which Virgil gathered his information]*, the great procession of the centuries is born anew...Now a new offspring is descending from high heaven...A race of gold shall arise throughout the world...Under their rule, Pollio *(sic)* shall this glorious age begin and the great months commence their progression...earth will pour forth her gifts without cultivation...The merchantmen shall retire from the sea...No longer shall earth suffer the harrow nor vines the pruning hook...See how the universe with its massive arch nods...See how all things rejoice in the age that is to come.''

The age that is to come is an image of the age that came before, the Ancient World, and as the human race of today approaches the same orientation of celestial influences which the people of the Ancient World shared, we begin to have the same mental images: we think in terms of the whole planet united in time of peace, creativity and harmony by the descending (centripetal) energy which formed the galaxy, the solar system, and this earth. That is the so-called Messianic age which began to be prophecied by spiritual leaders from 3,000 to 2,000 years ago as we entered the most recent stage in the polar cycle of 26,000 years—the transition period before the dawn.

Our vision of the future is based on our memory of the past. We assume the sun will come up tomorrow morning because it has always risen in a cycle of approximately 24 hours for as long as we can remember. Prophets like Isaiah or the author of the Book of Revelations were able to speak with authority of the Future World because their memories were large enough to encompass cycles like the one we have been examining. Let us now investigate some features of the Future World which we would expect to find on the basis of our memory of the Ancient World, aided by hints from the worldwide traditions of humanity.

The ancients apparently excelled people of the recent past in the faculties associated with ESP, teleportation, telekinesis, etc.; it seems they communicated with each other over great distances without using technological aids or material vehicles of transportation by tapping more profound and subtle forms of energy than we use in our material technology. Not only do traditional tales of flying and dematerialization and rematerialization suggest this superiority, but we also have the otherwise inexplicable remains of ancient constructions scattered from Peru to the Caucasus which contain massive hewn stones impossible to move by the most powerful modern machinery.

Aerial photographs also reveal huge networks of prehistoric highways that span the Amazon Basin. In order to understand why these ancient highways passed through what is now tropical jungle, we must study the displacement of climates caused by axis shifts which have recurred periodically throughout the earth's history.

When any object spins round and is itself somewhat elastic like the earth, it tends to broaden out at the equator due to the greater centrifugal force of rotation there. Eventually such spinning round objects become more and more disc-like. If you set an egg spinning on its flatter side, you will see how it rights itself to spin on end, in a manner similar to that which causes the periodic shifts in the earth's axis. Then the narrow equator starts to bulge again, and the whole process is repeated. Evidence for this having happened to the earth many times in the past comes from two kinds of physical evidence.

First, the magnetic orientation of igneous rocks which contain iron is not always found to point toward the present North Pole but varies systematically the deeper we probe into geological strata, indicating, for example, that the last South Pole was in Australia. Secondly, the world's great deserts do not occur regularly along the hottest portion of the globe, at the present equator where we would expect to find them, but instead stretch in a smoothly curving belt from the Gobi through the Sahara and down to South America (see Figure 5). The belt of deserts stretches along the former equator. Thus, the Amazon was formerly in a temperate zone, while the Atlantic coast of the United States had an arctic climate. Comparing the vegetation of the East Coast of the United States and the West Coast, we can see how much more luxurious and deep-rooted California trees, such as Sequoias and Redwoods are than anything comparable on the Atlantic. The soil of the Pacific Coast is much richer than the rocky ground of New England because the former was subject to a mild climate, similar to its present one, while the latter was covered by glacial ice.

Now we can begin to understand the basic but seemingly inexplicable cultural differences between civilization in the Eastern and Western Hemispheres. Until the last axis shift, roughly 13,000 years ago, Europe and Northeastern America (the cultural center of the occidental world) were relatively inhospitable territory, a cold land with shallow soil in which hard work and aggressiveness were necessities for survival.

A glance at Figure 5 shows that the Far East has had a relatively continuous history of comparative ease with much less dislocation in latitude than occurred in Europe because of the last axis shift. The East has not been obliged to rely on the hunting and animal husbandry that provide survival rations to maintain us in lands less suitable for the cultivation of cereal grains, humanity's staple food. The ecological capacity for a mainly vegetarian diet centered on grains and vegetables rather than animal food, plus the uninterrupted history of a relatively easy climate, has given the Orient its tranquil view of life.

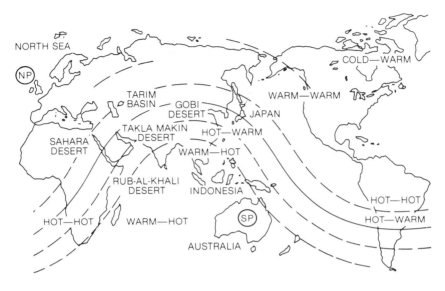

*Figure 5*

The famous, supposedly mystical, "Wisdom of the East" is the conse-
quence of natural factors. The relatively greater emphasis on spirit which
we associate with the East characterized, in fact, the civilization of the
Ancient World as a whole. Ever since the axis shift, however, the main
focus of activity has come increasingly from the West, which has
developed material technology, and the analytic mentality associated
with that technology, to great heights.

We are now witnessing a global meeting of East and West—holistic,
spiritual thought and analytical, scientific thought—as the pole star shifts
back toward its ancient location. The reconciliation of these two ways of
life will not represent the triumph of one over the other but a broader and
deeper synthesis of the strengths in each.

Technological civilization, at the extreme height of its development, is
now awakened to a concern for ecology, for example, that is based on
holistic rather than analytical ways of viewing the world.

In general, the simpler a technique, the greater its antiquity. In addition to so-called "paranormal" powers, in which the ancients excelled us
and to which we are reawakening, there is a growing appreciation for the
efficacy of natural ways in curing illness. The ancient method of treating
disease was not by surgery or medications, with all their complicated side

effects, but rather diet, massage, palm healing, and prayer. Prayer, in the sense of re-establishing our continuity with the infinite universe as the source of all life, was not then an esoteric profession assigned to an elite of spiritual technocrafts, as it has tended to be in the history of our institutionalized religions. It was the natural birthright of every human being, possessed—as the ancients were in full measure—of an intuitive ability to regain wholeness and health through self-reflection and reverent observation of nature. Nevertheless, there were also special centers, or shrines, where people could go to rededicate their energies and renew their mental and physical vitality. Even in historical times, the classical Greek center of healing at Epidaurus (sacred to Aesculapius, the god of medicine) was not only a place where the ailing went for simple physical treatments, such as herbs and baths, but was also a sacred site; the pa-

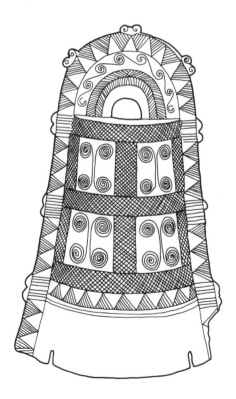

*Figure 6*

tients there fasted, slept in isolation in order to have dreams indicating the best method of cure, and witnessed dramatic performances in a natural setting which unified the restorative powers of poetry, theatre, music, and dance.

Not only the sense of place but also the sense of timing was extraordinarily important for the ancients living in close harmony with the cycles of nature. Throughout Asia archaeologists have found objects resembling a bell without a clapper (see Figure 6). These strange objects are pierced by two holes and marked on the inside with diagrams which specialists have not been able to decipher. If experiments were to be conducted seeing how light from the sun at critical times of the year, such as the summer and winter solstices, passes through those holes to shed its rays across the diagrams, these objects would be revealed as simple observatories. The most obvious value of such observational tools is the necessity for an agricultural community to know the best moments of planting and harvesting. The major monuments from the past—whether Stonehenge, the pyramids, the Mayan temples in Yucatan, or simple scratchings of five radiating lines found on boulders in the southwestern desert—have been shown to be precise astronomical tools for determining crucial agricultural times. In the next chapter we will see how a natural form of agriculture was the foundation of Ancient Civilization and must serve as our starting point for establishing global peace in the future world.

# 14

# The Future World

From the simple technology of a rude torch to drive away wild animals, on through the great empires of the Bronze Age based on smelting metals, and up to our own industrial civilization, fire has dominated the night side of the 25,800-year cycle discussed in the previous chapter. It has held the darkness at bay. Now, as the energy from our Milky Way Galaxy begins to revitalize the globe, our orientation can shift from the requisites of scarcity to the play of bounty. The primary cause of scarcity today—in the form of world-wide hunger, soil exhaustion, shortage of fuel, etc.—is the very technology we have developed to a point of diminishing returns. As our former ally, fire, becomes an enemy, our former enemy, the environment itself, becomes an ally.

The Dragon, feared so long in stories such as that of the Biblical serpent, now appears as a symbol for primary energy—alternating waves of natural change—honored among the most ancient cultures. The Dragon is a symbol of the Tao, which Lao Tsu compared to fire's opposite: "The highest goodness is like water, for water is excellent in benefiting all things and it does not strive." From the complex and the over-elaborated, we return to the simple and natural.

An awareness of this watershed quality to modern times motivates the current effort toward purification among many people now renewing their natural health. The natural lifestyle and natural foods movement is working to re-establish a sound physiological basis for humanity by dissolving the accumulated toxins from over-nutrition, excess medication, easy living—in short, spoiling. In the current epidemic increase of

Originally published in April, 1974 (East West Journal Vol. 4 No. 4)

chronic disease, the symptomatic treatments of modern medicine seem to cause more trouble than the problems they mean to remedy. What most patients need is not more treatment but a rational fast, not more prosperity but more contact with reality. People are setting out to unlearn the concepts they have been force-fed through education; they are replacing separation from nature and the panoply of fear with an intuitive appreciation for the basic justice of the universe.

The principles of paradise were expressed toward the beginning of this last, darkest period in the Great Year as the "Way of Nondoing" by Lao Tsu in the Orient, among others, or the Sermon on the Mount by Jesus in the West. These simple truths appear paradoxical only because we have been schooled in the conceptual modes of artificial thought separated from nature. In reality, the central corpus of spiritual truths are the most basic common sense.

That universal philosophy differs from conceptual ideas, which remain impractical abstractions, because it penetrates all aspects of life, including the biological foundation of our existence. People are now realizing that we cannot create peace on earth until we have revitalized the basis of our mental attitudes by a physiological change through our daily activity and diet. In order to restore the healthfulness of our food supply, however, we must transform our present agricultural methods.

A truly natural agriculture would return to the universal principle of balance which was used by humanity in its agriculture during the ancient period of Paradise. No agricultural implements have been found by archaeologists before 10,000 B.C.—i.e., 12,000 years ago, when the celestial North Pole was near Vega and the Paradise half of the Great Year turned into the laborious half. The absence of plows, axes, pruning hooks, hoes, etc. does not mean that there was no agriculture in the Ancient Garden of Eden, but that agriculture was not conducted with the violent methods to which we have grown accustomed.

When we have grown blind to wholeness and can no longer see every process as a balanced cycle, when we can't remember a clear dream of the future, we resort to expediency. Through fear we have changed the surface of the earth, striving to ensure a good harvest; the cause of fear is lack of faith.

Approaches based on fear—most obvious in the modern applied sciences of medicine—treat symptoms as problems to be corrected, rather than understanding the necessary part they play in the whole system. Let's see how this kind of violent, fearful thinking operates in agriculture.

The first thing a farmer does when he goes to the country is to cut down the trees, so his crops receive more sunlight. Losing more water through greater evaporation in the sun, the plants now need irrigation. Then the resulting large, watery plants growing on the area of land need fertilizer to maintain the concentration of available minerals in their systems which now is low, relative to their artificially supplemented water content. Therefore farmers spread fertilizer, which is heavy work, but now at last the plants are big and rich in minerals! But how tempting to all the so-called harmful bacteria and insect pests. Out come the pesticides, which inconveniently kill the beneficial bugs as well. There seems no end to it.

When any farm is started, two basic principles are taken for granted. First, remove all weeds. Second, segregate crops into different areas. The end results of these normally unquestioned procedures are disease in the food crops (and therefore in man) and endless work.

We start out, in other words, by removing "undesirable" realities to arm's length and then keeping what's left in separate compartments for the sake of efficiency through mass production. Segregating crops into different fields robs them of the natural chemical as well as electromagnetic complementary balances which they receive when growing together in the wild. In the same way, modern civilization tends to isolate artists from scientists, laborers from businessmen, etc. in different neighborhoods and subcultures to their great mutual impoverishment. Since we have been creating our bodies and nervous systems from weakened foods, which are the distorted products of artificial agriculture, we have lost our mental clarity and are unable to see the utter folly of our unnatural farming methods.

In holistic rather than analytic terms, what is the food that we get from plants? The grains and the fruit are the portion for reproduction remaining after the cycle of the plant's metabolism has been balanced between internal production and internal consumption. When we stimulate a plant's internal system of production, we also stimulate its consumption, and the net result is zero—if we take care to consider the quality as well as the quantity of the resulting food.

Many people now know how much better an organic vegetable tastes than a chemicalized one, but how many of us have tasted a wild carrot?

Probably we wouldn't even like it so much at first—too strong. It's been able to survive among weeds, so it wasn't over-fed and protected. Just imagine what exciting lives, what intimate harmony with nature, what powerful intuition we could have if we lived off truly natural food.

The ancient method of natural agriculture may look impractical at first sight but only because moderns have no experience of a natural life. In fact, nothing could be easier. The entire method can be described in the following points:

1. If weeds are growing on a site, we can use it, since plants already have survived there. Only if no weeds grow—such as on rocky hills—should we leave that area alone.
2. Don't remove any weeds before sowing.
3. Don't plough or till the soil.
4. Don't separate crops into different areas.
5. Use minimum fertilization by domestic animals and by strictly local mulching. If we want to, and just for the first year, we can remove weeds in the fall and dry them over the winter for use as mulch to protect our first sowing from being eaten by the birds.
6. Give very careful attention to the proper time for sowing. Sow summer and fall vegetables at that period in the spring when winter weeds have begun to die and before spring weeds have started up. Then sow your winter and spring vegetables when summer weeds are withering and fall weeds haven't sprung up yet. Always plant just before the rain.
7. Don't plant seeds, dropping them in a hole and then covering it over. The plants in nature grow quite well by going to seed without any farmer burying them when they fall to the ground. Through timing alone, the drying weeds and the rain will cover the seeds we sow sufficiently.

   People started burying seeds in the ground after the great error of weeding had been instituted. In fact the weeds secure soil porosity for the descending roots of new plants as well as fostering the presence of beneficial bacteria.

   Don't forget to sow many different kinds of vegetables together in the same area. Thus the soil will never be depleted in any one particular mineral. This practice also serves to keep away animal pests, which will be repelled by the odors and the visible as well as invisible radiant energies of the complementary plants scattered among whatever vegetables a particular animal or insect is attracted to.

8. If we choose land that is heavily forested, our logging should be kept to a minimum. Thin a little, but not just one species or size. From two acres we'll have enough wood to build our homes.

Since our naturally grown food will be very nutritious and concentrated, there will be more than enough land to support the population of the earth, and then some. The birth rate will also return to reflecting the natural cycles of scarcity and abundance in the food we eat. In accord with the natural sequence of lean and plentiful harvests, an annually varying probability for conceiving and giving birth will reflect these alternating high and low levels of metabolic excess available for reproduction.

Before the Fall under Vega, humanity must have lived not in villages or cities but in simple hut-like constructions in the forest land. Civilization as we know it throughout recorded history since the Bronze Age is identical with the separation of city and country—places of food consumption and food production. This division is the beginning of commerce and, of course, large-scale transportation. The culmination of this alienating system is the modern megalopolis. The foundations for the schizophrenia of modern society were dug with the first systematic farm.

As we create a sound biological basis for our lives, the delusive concepts of our artificial civilization will disperse like the phantoms of a dream. People in the future will wonder how anyone could have seriously believed that one view is right and all others are wrong, that power can create justice, that analysis can reveal truth, that medicine can cure illness, or that nations really exist and can demand the sacrifice of our lives. Where is the basis in reality for these groundless concepts that we have learned to take for granted?

National boundaries, for example, have no real existence outside our conceptual minds; we have hypnotized ourselves to think that the map's different colors somehow prevail on the actual earth. Fortunately, the animals and the seeds carried on the wind have not attended any classes in citizenship. Our descendants will have no word for freedom because they will be free. Our present freedom is the right to obtain passports, visas, marriage licenses, etc. and to pay for what belongs to no one. What does a Justice of the Peace, for example, have to do with two people's desire to build their lives together? No religions will exist in the future either, for spirituality will be an ordinary part of daily life, as we naturally remember our oneness with the environing total universe. The basic necessities of life belong to everyone. How can food or land ever be paid for, when they come from the universe as the air and the sunlight? Shall we pay rent in the womb?

Ecological areas do exist, of course, but different from national territories in that the latter are artificial. That's why the state must be maintained by force—not only the obvious forms of power in armies and allied industries but also the even more destructive form of violence called mass education.

We all have passed at least 10 to 20 years of our lives in the task of strangling our natural intelligence. Has anything we learned at school helped us to live more wisely or really more usefully? Something is false at the root of a society which demands this wasteful indoctrination in abstract knowledge as a prerequisite for respected membership. Of all the damage perpetrated by those who claim to know what's best for us, the greatest by far is done by teachers. A true teacher is himself or herself an embodiment of the Tao, serving as an example of living in continuity with the spontaneous order of the universe, just as a real doctor must be a vibrantly healthy person. In the future people will find it hard to believe that we relied on doctors who could not cure themselves.

Young people are increasingly aware of how much healthier organic and so-called natural foods are than commercial, mass-produced fare. But so long as this movement is motivated by the rudimentary desire for physical health alone, it still belongs to the mentality of scarcity-orientation and isolated security. "Organic food is good for you" is merely a switch in terms from "meat is good for you;" it is not a change in basic mentality. We have pushed open the doors of our prison cells but still linger inside.

People who used to say, for example, "I want some ice cream," after they ate a steak now say, "I'd like some apple pie made with maple syrup," after they've had some miso soup. But that illusory "I" is still taken with total seriousness. In actuality, it's the saltiness of steak or miso soup that requires something sweet as balance; the salt in us is what wants dessert. We assume that we ourselves pick out from the world whatever objects we select for food, but we only have the illusion of *taking*: the particular food that already forms our bodies and mental state *attracts* another food, its complement. The "I" is a concept as completely fictional as national boundaries.

We can see Buddha, Lao Tsu, and other great spiritual leaders as revolutionaries demolishing this most powerful of all unnecessary institutions: the ego—the fiction that we are somehow radically separate from the universe. Real freedom is not any political security, the insurance that our birthright will be stolen from us according to law. Nor, on the other hand, does it come by political revolution, seizing control from those in power. There's no need to defend or overturn the system violently, for under the Milky Way's rain of energy only those will be able to function effectively who can follow the path of emptiness.

Yin fosters yang, and yang leads to yin; weakness elicits strength and strength ends in weakness. By accumulating strength we eventually grow spoiled; by cultivating humility, modesty, and emptiness we become clear channels for the primary energy that is now descending upon the earth from The Milky Way overhead, and ultimately from the cosmic plenum which formed our galaxy.

Primitive is not always the same as natural. The primitive food gatherer under Hercules who thoroughly exhausted one area and then moved on to another differs in lack of sophistication but not in his basic philosophy from the modern industrialist or agribusinessman functioning under Polaris. The essence of natural agriculture is using nature freely but with wisdom, understanding her laws of perennial balance. We can have a technology vastly superior to the present cumbersome system, when we have learned to work in harmony with those universal principles.

The obsolescence of governments that presume to regulate our lives does not mean there will be no unifying centers in the future. True government serves to offer information (such as the best time for planting, harvesting, etc.), to receive the suggestions of everyone, and to plan festivities that reunite humanity with Heaven and Earth. Under the influence of the Milky Way directly over the North Pole people will not only consume less but will need less sleep. There will be festivals for the full moon, the new moon, and perhaps the half and the crescent! We have difficulty imagining our ancient and future capacity for play, because we are trained in the ethos of drudgery. People once celebrated and will again honor the blooming of new flowers. Every such gathering dances to the silent music of the spheres. The reborn art of the ancients will put our conceptual efforts to shame: appreciating emptiness, the void moving with infinite possibilities, the beauty of their poetry lies not in the individual words but in the intervals between. In their painting, preserved for us in caves and on rocks, we glimpse the primacy of space over the material objects which emerge from it.

That is the peaceful yet dynamic world we are creating, and calculated plans to survive the present chaos in isolated security are what we've had too much of. The future is created not through any social engineering nor by waiting until we finally know enough to act without mistakes. We create the future right now by the way we eat every day, by the way we greet each other, by taking off our shoes in the evening and placing one beside the other for our children to see as a wordless example of orderly living. If we live our daily lives in that spirit of balance, we don't have to worry about the future; it will appear because we made room for it.

Like vibrant seeds we must be "lean and hungry." The realization of our dream depends on the sureness of our appetite, both physical and spiritual. The modern world never lets us get really hungry for anything, and that's the greatest exploitation of all—the spiritual deprivation that comes from having perfected the art of taking, of filling ourselves. Love however is endless, because it is giving—an emptying of oneself that is forever replenished.

A new Orpheus will rejoin Eurydice, the Spinning Maid will cross the bridge of the Milky Way to her lover once more—and then the couples must separate, but they can never forget. Infinity is One through continual balance, unchanging change. The force of Heaven descends as the spirit of Earth rises with us to build One Peaceful World again.

*East West Journal,* one of the nation's principal magazines advocating the importance of a healthful diet, has been published for fourteen years from Brookline, Massachusetts. Long before it became fashionable to dine on granola, yoghurt, and tofu, *East West Journal* was stressing the value of eating less saturated fats and more fiber and complex carbohydrates. The value of eating whole and natural foods is one of the primary topics of every issue of *EWJ*.

This magazine will show you how to eat better and live longer and more healthfully—but you may have to cut your food bill in half to do so. We'll show you how to do it the way the U.S. Government's Dietary Guidelines recently recommended: With whole grains and fiber and a healthful alternative to the standard American diet.

*East West Journal* is a magazine with an objective: The holistic quality of life...physical, spiritual, and intellectual.

The writers of the *Journal* are people you can trust and rely on. They are people who have made a natural lifestyle their lifestyle. And they write on everything from organic gardening, wilderness trekking, and long distance running, to spinning yarn, making your own pickles, and raising children naturally.

The issue of diet is always part of *East West Journal.* But it's only one part. Each issue of *EWJ* is as eclectic as the holistic view we take of the world. You'll find regular columns on natural healing, ecology, alternative energy, family health, books, and natural foods cooking.

*EWJ* is available in selected natural foods stores and bookstores throughout the U.S. and Europe. Subscriptions are available for only $18.00 for one year. Please address your subscription order to *East West Journal* P.O. Box 1200, Department W, 17 Station Street, Brookline, Massachusetts 02147.